LIVING LONGER

IN THE *BOOMER AGE*

COMBINING ALTERNATIVE AND CONVENTIONAL MEDICINE FOR MAXIMUM HEALTH AND VITALITY

JOHN L. ZENK, M.D.

Advanced
Research Press

New York 1998

For information contact: Advanced Research Press, Inc., 150 Motor Pkwy., Suite 210, Hauppauge, New York 11788.

FIRST EDITION

Library of Congress Catalog-in-Publication Data

1. Health

2. Title

ISBN 1-889462-03-9

Printed in the United States of America

Published by: **Advanced Research Press**
150 Motor Pkwy.
Suite 210
Hauppauge, New York 11788

Publisher/President: Steve Blechman

Project Director: Roy Ulin

Art Director: Rob Wilner (DotCom)

Cover Design: Sam Powell

Copy Editing: Advanced Research Press Staff

Printed by: DotCom

Dedication

I dedicate this book to Neal Richards, whose personal strength, perseverance and undying optimism are a shining example to spinal cord injured people everywhere, and for that matter, the entire human race.

John L. Zenk, MD

John started his professional career as a pharmacist completing his training at the University of Minnesota-College of Pharmacy in 1978. He was employed as a hospital pharmacist at United Hospital in St. Paul, MN for one year. He was very active in teaching pharmacy students for the University of Minnesota during that time. He then entered the University of Minnesota-Medical School where he completed his MD training and was elected to the Alpha Omega Alpha National Medical Honor Society for his academic excellence during those four years. He chose Internal Medicine as his specialty and completed his three year residency at the Hennepin County Medical Center in Minneapolis in 1986.

After residency and becoming Board Certified in Internal Medicine, John pursued his first full time medical position at the Hutchinson Medical Center in Hutchinson, MN. While at Hutchinson, John was the Medical Director of the Intensive and Coronary Care Unit at the local hospital in addition to being Chief of Staff for four years. He also spent nine years as the Director of Emergency Medical Services. John continued his passion for teaching students and while at Hutchinson became a Clinical Assistant Professor of Medicine at the University of Minnesota-Medical School, because of his excellent reputation with medical students.

John's experience in Hutchinson was quite fulfilling as a medical doctor. He spearheaded many new programs at the Hutchinson Community Hospital including a complete hemodynamic monitoring system for the ICU, a "Trauma

Code" program, a team oriented plan for the resuscitation of severely injured trauma patients entering the ER which was very successful. He implanted the first dual chamber permanent cardiac pacemaker in a patient at that hospital in addition to performing over 5000 gastrointestinal endoscopy procedures. He was Chairman of their Total Quality Management Team and the Director of the Cardiac Rehabilitation Program.

After leaving Hutchinson, John accepted a position at the St. Francis Regional Medical Center in Shakopee, MN. There he was Chief of Medicine and served as the Director of Intensive and Coronary Care. He also was Chairman and Director of the Cardiac Care Center at St. Francis. Both in Hutchinson and Shakopee, John has maintained a very active and loyal outpatient clinical practice as well.

John's career has now taken him to a new position with an independent group of Internists called Internal Medicine and Geriatric Associates, Inc. He practices out of Fairview Riverside and Abbott Northwestern Hospitals in Minneapolis.

John remains quite active in a number of national and local associations and organizations including: American Medical Association, Minnesota Medical Association, Hennepin County Medical Society, The American College of Physicians, American Society of Internal Medicine, and the Society of General Internal Medicine to name a few.

Contents

Preface

During the early years of my practice in conventional medicine, I thought I could solve most of my patients' ailments, and that allopathic medicine had all the answers. As you will realize as you read this book, conventional medicine does not have all the answers and there are a number of afflictions, particularly chronic diseases, which respond just as well to complementary (or alternative) therapies. The movement toward complementary medical practices, which is developing across this country, is testament to the fact that these therapies are effective and that the public is demanding them as part of their overall treatment plan.

I believe therefore that it is finally time, after hundreds of years of medical practice, both conventional and complementary, for an integration process to take place. The integration of conventional medical practice with complementary medicine represents a new way of thinking about modern health care delivery - what I call the BoomerAge Model. This model gives patients more options for relief of their symptoms.

Baby boomers ("Boomers") are the driving force behind this concept. Boomers represent a population of 80 million people born between 1946 and 1964. They have been a formidable group of people who have single-handedly changed the course of history. Since I am a member of this group, I can testify to the fact that everything from automobiles to electronic equipment and fast foods have evolved and become a lasting part of our lives because of the Boomers' ideas and desires. They now are having an impact on the way we practice medicine.

As a group, Boomers question and challenge everything. Nothing to them is black and white. If it can be done another way, Boomers have found it. In my practice, most Boomers have questioned conventional healing methods and have sought relief of their problems from alternative practitioners or herbal therapies. They have challenged me to think with an open-mind and to consider more than just conventional health practices to heal their diseases. Interestingly, as you will read later in the book, the process of integrating conventional medicine with alternative medicine has worked for many of my own patients and hundreds of others.

Boomers as a group feel that taking an active role in their own health care has given them more control of their outcomes and has allowed them to feel better faster. This is a concept that I whole-heartedly support based on observations that whenever patients are engaged with their care plan, they are more compliant and mentally driven toward an accelerated healing course. Once again Boomers are right and will no doubt change the course of history.

This book is therefore different than most you will read on the topic of alternative health practices or dietary supplements. The BoomerAge Model promotes the integration of conventional and alternative medicine, not just the use of alternative medical practices alone. Since many alternative medical practices have not been subjected to the rigors of conventional medical efficacy studies, i.e. double-blind placebo controlled studies, they should only be used in consultation with a health practitioner.

The BoomerAge Model promotes practitioner-guided use of dietary supplements and alternative health practices when approaching the treatment of a disease. This model also urges companies to provide scientific support for new dietary ingredients. This includes conducting appropriate safety and efficacy studies to help the public and health practitioners know what these new compounds will do and what side effects they are likely to encounter.

The BoomerAge Model may require that conventional physicians learn more about the benefits of integrating these two methods of health care. I am sure there will be the expected amount of resistance to this concept, but again, the Boomers will drive this process. They will get advice from their physicians or seek out other "complementary-friendly" doctors who will help them. Economically, this could have enormous impact on managed care systems that may restrict their physicians to conventional practice. It is essential that health practitioners listen to their patient's ideas and opinions regarding complementary therapies.

A good example of complementary therapy is DHEA. Since the introduction of DHEA as a dietary supplement in 1995, there has been much media attention on its use and health benefits. This book will introduce you to a promising new metabolic analog of DHEA called 7-Keto DHEA. 7-Keto DHEA is now available under the Twinlab MaxiLIFE™ 7-Keto and Twinlab 7-Keto Fuel™ brands in health food stores as a new dietary supplement. 7-Keto DHEA is particularly exciting, since it provides enhanced benefits of DHEA without increasing sex hormones.

As appropriate background information, we will discuss

the human endocrine system as it relates to our natural hormone function. Also, we will review the parent compound DHEA. Finally, I will introduce you to a new phenomenon occurring in the dietary supplement industry. A phenomenon that I believe represents a new frontier for that industry.

This new frontier involves creating new products from existing naturally occurring substances, by finding metabolic derivatives of their parent compounds. The pharmaceutical industry has been taking advantage of this process for years, and now the dietary supplement industry has their chance to introduce many new and promising compounds to the market. DHEA derivatives are just the beginning, and since many researchers are focused in this area, many other compounds will certainly follow.

The introduction of 7-Keto DHEA represents the first commercial introduction of a metabolic derivative of a naturally occurring substance to the dietary supplement industry. Restoring youthful levels of a naturally occurring hormone in the human body makes obvious sense. There are pre-clinical and clinical safety studies to support its use.

Benefits of 7-Keto DHEA include an improvement in cognitive alertness and "revving" up the human immune system. Boomers will find it an aid to relieving stress and fatigue, particularly in women. Other benefits are discussed later in this book and are equally promising.

I believe much attention will be given to this new supplement and the public will greatly benefit. 7-Keto DHEA is more potent than its parent, DHEA, and it cannot be converted to sex hormones.

Please read this book with an open mind and form your

own conclusions about the BoomerAge Model, the future of complementary medical practices and the responsible use of dietary supplements. Also, as you read, please refer to the back of the book for a listing of references used to document the information needed to write this book. In addition, there is a glossary for understanding the definitions of certain medical terms.

John L. Zenk, M.D.

CHAPTER ONE

The Myth of Conventional Medicine

As a conventional medical doctor, I have diagnosed and treated thousands of patients over the years. Contrary to popular belief, I have found that not all treatments using conventional medicine are effective and that patients react differently to similar therapies.

As a former pharmacist, I also realized long ago that conventional allopathic medicine, although deeply woven into the academy of the healing arts, and trusted by many, does not have all the answers, nor should it be depended upon as the only treatment for certain diseases. In fact, I see a movement developing across this country suggesting, and in some cases demanding, that health care providers incorporate complementary medical practices into the therapy of patients with diseases not responding to conventional therapies.

I have experienced this in my own practice and have watched it evolve in my colleagues' practices as well. My experience as a medical doctor includes 14 years as a general internist with a practice emphasis in cardiovascular diseases and critical care. This type of practice, over the years, has developed into a life of taking care of intensely sick people, most of whom are elderly. My current practice has also evolved into one that has an emphasis on chronic diseases, many of which have no cure.

My job has been to make these people as comfortable as possible with their diseases, realizing that they have few, if any, effective treatment options. Over time, with any one given patient, my treatment armamentarium grows smaller and smaller until I have very little left to offer them. I have discovered that when I incorporate complementary medical options into my treatment plans, I have more to offer my patients and they often appreciate these therapies, since they usually have more of a personal touch.

What I eventually discovered was that my patients were seeking out complementary medical treatment modalities on their own, paying for them out of their own pockets and reporting back to me that the results were good. In many cases, these patients were totally healed of their ailment. The concept of a patient reporting their personal findings to their doctor was unheard of three years ago. It was not until I began to share my interest in their personal struggles to treat their diseases that they began to share their stories with me.

I found all this very intriguing, since the interactions seemed to improve our doctor/patient relationship. Many of my patients began sending me books and tapes on various complementary treatment modalities. I then began routinely incorporating complementary therapies into my treatment regimens. The results are promising, and better yet, my patients are more involved than ever in their treatment plans.

This is something I have been trying to improve on since I took the Hippocratic Oath. There appears to be a new model for health care developing where the consumer desires that his or her health care provider utilize all acceptable and safe treatment options when treating their disease, whether they are conventional and allopathic or non-conventional and complementary.

According to government reports, improving the health

status of the United States citizens ranks at the top of the national priorities of the Federal Government. Their reports go on to cite that the importance of nutrition and the benefits of dietary supplements to health promotion and disease prevention have been documented increasingly in scientific studies.

There also appears to be a link between ingestion of certain nutrients, or dietary supplements, and the prevention of chronic diseases such as cancer, heart disease and osteoporosis. National surveys have revealed that almost 50 percent of the 260 million Americans regularly consume dietary supplements of vitamins, minerals or herbs as a means of improving their nutrition. Other studies indicate that consumers are placing increased reliance on the use of complementary health care providers to avoid the excessive cost of conventional medical services, and to obtain more holistic consideration of their needs.

These statistics scare me since I know from my own practice experience, that many of these people are taking dietary supplements without knowing anything about them or their side effects. For instance, some patients are achieving good results with herbal therapy while others are disappointed. An integrated model using the physicians to help guide therapy is the obvious answer to this dilemma. It would help save patients time and money, and promote healing using conventional and when appropriate, complementary therapies.

The Dietary Supplement Health and Education Act (DSHEA) was passed in 1994 in response to the growing desire of consumers to learn more about and begin practicing preventive health care. This includes diet, nutrition and the appropriate use of safe dietary supplements to help reduce the potential of chronic diseases. The Act creates a new framework for the regulation of dietary supplements by the Secretary of the Department of Health and Human Services and is premised on the role of nutrition and the benefits of dietary supplements in health promotion. The Act also reaffirms the status of dietary supplements as foods and creates a new dietary supplement category that includes vitamins, minerals, herbs or other botanicals, amino acids and other dietary substances.

The Act has opened the door to the introduction of many new dietary supplements to the market. In addition, metabolites or extracts of these dietary ingredients can also be marketed as dietary supplements. Many researchers have been waiting for this opportunity to introduce safe new dietary ingredients. With the aid of the Boomers demanding more therapeutic options, this field of research will flourish.

Therefore, based on my own personal practice experiences, and the position of the United States Government on these issues, I believe it behooves all of us to take a close look at the latest research and literature on the subject of dietary supplements and their role as therapeutic agents.

We should also be looking to the dietary supplement industry to provide and adhere to standards of excellence that exceed the requirements of the DSHEA. As more and more consumers begin to utilize dietary supplements as part of their care plan, there will be an obvious need to assure the public that what they are buying is what is printed on the label.

Also, as more and more physicians begin to support the

use of dietary supplements there will be an even greater need for higher purity standards and accurate safety data on these supplements. Eventually as these supplements become more sophisticated and a part of any patient's treatment plan, I believe the need for valid efficacy studies will intensify at the urging of Boomers and their doctors.

The BoomerAge Model supports the use of dietary supplements and urges an integration of conventional and complementary care for the benefit of patients. The model encourages conventional physicians to educate themselves about complementary health practices and then guide their patients in their quest for and use of dietary supplements and other complementary treatment modalities. This model therefore fosters the use of both conventional and complementary medical practices, providing they are safe and that they help patients feel better.

The next chapter describes some of my early experiences with complementary medicine in my practice. I hope it also provides a basis for discussing the practical applications of the BoomerAge Model in any primary care medical practice.

Convincing A Skeptic

It wasn't that long ago when I would have rejected the idea of using complementary medicine in my practice. In fact, when I was practicing in a rural community in central Minnesota during my early years in practice, I was challenged by my medical colleagues for referring patients to chiropractors for help with their back pain. They said that the chiropractors were charlatans and "quacks," and that they should not be trusted. Nonetheless, my patients went to them on their own or at my advice and got relief of their symptoms. My father, who has had a painful lower back and hip most of his life, swears by his chiropractic treatments and visited his chiropractor quite often while I was growing up.

Gradually my opinions about complementary therapy began to change, and I would have to say that my patients, not the medical community, convinced me to consider it as part of my practice. One example of this that really changed my mind occurred in 1992 with one of my patients, and I will call her "Patty." Patty said I could use her story in this book.

Patty was 52 years old when she came to my clinic one day complaining that she was experiencing moderate to severe pain all over her body. The pain was not localized to any particular area, nor was it involving her joints, but rather was in her muscles and areas near joints. The pain was interfering with her lifestyle and her sleep, and, in fact, her normal sleep cycle was quite disrupted. She was waking up numerous times during the night, and awoke every morning feeling tired and in pain. This seemed to be a vicious cycle for her and she was desperate for relief. She denied any recent trauma or other illnesses that were affecting her concomitantly.

Patty's physical examination was nearly normal, except for several symmetric trigger points of pain, which I could elicit by pressing on them. In fact, this examination maneuver was able to reproduce the pain she was having almost exactly. We found no evidence for active arthritis in any of her joints and no evidence for other disease.

We, of course, next did a thorough lab work-up and some x-rays, but again found no clear evidence for collagen vascular diseases such as lupus and no other diagnoses surfaced as the lab work was reviewed.

After reviewing the results of the labs and reviewing her physical findings, which persisted, the diagnosis was clear. Patty had fibromyalgia, also called fibrositis. This disease affects the connective tissues of the body, and as a result, a severe inflammatory response arises. We, in the conventional medical community, believe that fibromyalgia/fibrositis is precipitated and eventually sustained because of the disruption in the sleep cycle[1]. We believe that if patients do not obtain Stage III and Stage IV sleep (these are the deepest stages of sleep), that their connective tissues will not be allowed to maintain themselves, and eventually they will begin to hurt as a result of this neglect.

Patty seemed to understand and was hopeful that if I could restore her sleep cycle that her pain would disappear. I, of course, was also hopeful since I had treated many patients before her and had achieved excellent results with most of them using a therapy which restores the sleep cycle.

---

[1] Please refer to the glossary in the back for an understanding of the medical terminology used in this book.

So, Patty and I embarked on a treatment plan which included the use of a drug called Amitriptyline, which is actually an anti-depressant medication, but has remarkable sedating qualities to it. Patty followed my instructions to the letter and we started out at 50 mg at bedtime and eventually increased to 100 mg every night. The drug worked very well and she slept great for about two and a half months.

Normally, this type of response should result in an improvement in the symptoms of fibromyalgia, but much to my disbelief, Patty was as miserable as ever and complained of the same pain. I was frustrated because I knew if restoring the sleep cycle was ineffective that I did not have much else to offer her. Patty and I decided to try other sleeping medications, anti-inflammatory medications and physical therapy.

She was in my clinic almost weekly and I felt sorry for her since she was not getting any better. Everything I had tried had failed. This went on for nearly six months and at the end of a very rigorous treatment trial, Patty had chronic pain that was destroying her life. In fact, she had lost her job and rarely socialized outside of her home.

I suggested to her that in the absence of any good treatments to this point that I had to consider this a chronic fibromyalgia syndrome, and that she should begin attending the Fibromyalgia Support Group in our city to better learn how to live with the disease.

Patty thought this was a good idea and attended several meetings. In fact, I was asked to speak to the group on a number of occasions and met several people like Patty who had chronic fibromyalgia. The group was good for Patty, and by making contact with others who had her disease, she no longer felt alone, being better able to cope.

Patty was still coming into my clinic for treatment, but not as frequently. After she did not return for six months, I presumed she was still in pain and coping with the help of her friends.

Finally Patty returned to see me, but this time, something was different. She was smiling! She had bought new clothes, was active and did not appear to be in pain. I said, "Patty, how are you? You look healthy and happy." She replied, "Dr. Zenk, I feel terrific! My pain is gone and I am getting my life back together."

"That's wonderful!" I said, "What happened that changed your life?" She then went on to tell me that during one of their support group meetings a local herbalist had come to talk to them. She was impressed with what he had to say at the meeting and later contacted him on her own to discuss her case.

The two of them embarked on a new treatment plan that included two different herbal treatments, along with some vitamin and mineral supplements. Her pain was controlled with a separate herbal therapy, which worked well to keep her comfortable. Patty took the regimen for two months, paid for it out of her own pocket, and told me nothing about it until after six months had passed. She reported that over the previous two months, she could feel her body rejuvenating until one day, her pain was gone completely and she could go through an entire day without even thinking about her ailment. She was a new person!

I was overjoyed; she looked so healthy, I couldn't believe it! To this day she comes to my clinic about every six months, continues to take a maintenance dosage of her treatment and feels fine. She also related her experiences to the rest of her group, and many of them escaped their misery as well.

This enlightening case changed my life and I began to research complementary therapies for other chronic diseases I was seeing in my clinic. The BoomerAge Model started to become a reality for me. It was in its infancy at that point, in my mind, and I started to wonder what would happen if I integrated my conventional treatments with my new found complementary treatments.

I began to realize that conventional medicine did not have adequate treatments for a lot of my patients with chronic diseases. I made some early internal inquires about complementary medicine in my practice and found that it was very popular with my patients. I then decided to begin a more formal survey of my practice and eventually interviewed 200 of my patients on this subject. What I found was truly enlightening and convinced me that the idea of integrating conventional and complementary medical practices had merit, the BoomerAge Model started to take shape.

The results of my survey revealed that in 1993, 160 patients, or 80 percent of those 200 patients, were using some form of complementary medicine. 63 percent of the patients had one or more chronic disease. 65 percent of these patients reported an improvement in their condition with these therapies. (See Figure 1 for a list of the diseases that these patients had and see Figure 2 for a listing of the various complementary therapies I asked about in the survey.) 70 percent of these patients had not told me anything about their use of these therapies. All therapies were paid for out-of-pocket and were not covered by insurance. 40 percent of these patients had sought help with their therapy decisions via books and other written reference material, and 60 percent took the advice of friends, relatives or providers of these therapies.

Patients' Diseases
 Chronic pain
 Chronic fatigue syndrome
 Cancer
 Arthritis
 Eating disorders
 Irritable bowel syndrome
 AIDS
 Habit control
 Chronic renal failure
 Fibromyalgia/fibrositis
 Neurologic conditions such as Bell's Palsy

Figure 1.

Patients' Complementary Therapies
   Chiropractic
   Acupuncture
   Biofeedback
   Homeopathy
   Massage
   Herbalism
   Hypnosis
   Psychospiritual
   Nutritional aids
   Vitamin therapy
   Macrobiotics

Figure 2.

After the survey was complete, I was convinced that the BoomerAge Model of integrating health care had merit and I wanted to know more about complementary health practices and what they could do for my patients. During the next six months I researched the various aspects of complementary health practices. I quickly realized that there was an active movement developing across the country embracing complementary medicine.

There were a lot of skeptics, but nonetheless, it was becoming clear that patients wanted better access to these therapies, and wanting their physicians to become more knowledgeable on the subject and help them with their decisions.

I found that several important events occurred in the early and mid-1990's to start this movement rolling. The first and probably most important event was the publishing of Dr. Richard Eisenberg's study in the *New England Journal of*

Medicine in January 1993. This is one of traditional medicine's most prestigious and well-read medical journals, and in a hurry, got everyone thinking more seriously about complementary medicine.

Dr. Eisenberg's study revealed that one-third of all Americans were seeking out complementary medicine, and the number of visits to nontraditional providers of care out-numbered visits to traditional doctors (425 million visits versus 388 million visits). The study also revealed findings similar to my own, in that 72 percent of patients had not told their physicians they were using these therapies. The majority of them paid for it out of their own pockets.

Probably the most startling statistic to me was that these Americans spent **$13.7 billion** on complementary treatments of all kinds. The highest use was among people ages 25 to 49 (the Boomers). They belonged to higher education and higher income brackets throughout the country. Dr. Eisenberg concluded that physicians should ask their patients about the use of complementary medicine.

The Eisenberg movement, as I like to call it, soon swept the country and it was not long before the National Institutes of Health (NIH) established the Office of Alternative Medicine (OAM), aimed at investigation of the field. The OAM will be studying seven different categories of alternative care. These are: mind/body interventions; bio-electromagnetic therapies; alternative systems of medical practice; manual healing methods; pharmacologic and biologic treatments; herbal medicine; and diet and nutrition.

The OAM has a modest federal budget and currently has set numerous study sites across the country to investigate these treatments. Their results should be very thought-provoking.

The Dietary Supplement Health and Education Act of 1994 was then passed by our lawmakers. This act places vitamins, herbs, minerals and naturally occurring substances in a category all their own as dietary supplements, not drugs. This allows more of these therapeutic substances to be introduced to the market and be available to the public.

The *Journal of the American Board of Family Practice* published an article in 1995 revealing that 70 to 90 percent of physicians considered complementary medical therapies to be legitimate medical practices. The majority of the physicians had made referrals for these therapies. The physicians surveyed felt that the specialties within complementary care with little or no training were less legitimate.

The Eisenberg movement eventually hit the media and it is to the point now that nearly every magazine you pick up has an article about complementary medicine. Not to mention the coverage of the topic on the major television news programs educating us about the virtues of complementary care. Numerous books have been written based on the movement as well, with Dr. Andrew Weil as a prominent and inspirational author. My local newspaper in Minneapolis also frequently reports on complementary medical topics of interest.

Lastly, I have learned the most from my patients who now regularly send me books, cassette tapes, videos and other written material on what they are trying. It seems that since I have shown an interest in their desire to use these therapies, they are increasingly willing to share their ideas, treatment regimens and results with me, a move which has really brought all of us closer together and working as a team to make them healthy.

Therefore, after many months—and now years—of research, it is quite clear to me that the use of complementary medical therapies should be integrated into existing conventional practices. It is my hope that managed care organizations and insurance companies will embrace this integration process, allowing patients to receive these therapies as part of their normal treatment protocol and as a natural part of their health plan premium. Some of this is already happening in select areas of the United States.

With this information in hand, I began integrating complementary medical therapies into my own practice. I have found them to be quite useful and my patients loved it. Some of the changes I have made in my practice include asking as part of my normal history-taking process a question about their use of complementary medicine. I then know they are interested in these therapies and they know that I am cognizant of complementary care. For chronic diseases, in particular, I now give my patients the option of conventional care and conventional care integrated with complementary care.

Once the decision to pursue complementary care is made, I either refer them to complementary providers for acupuncture or other treatments, or I give them handouts with complementary treatment ideas for their specific disease that they can pursue on their own.

This integration has given me more treatment options for many chronic diseases and has decreased utilization of conventional services, which is certainly a benefit in a capitated medical delivery system. This integration has also been helpful in allowing me to know everything my patient is taking. Many times this has influenced my decisions regarding their conventional treatment programs.

For instance, if I know one of my patients is going to a chiropractor and getting manipulation and acupuncture, I will withhold sending them to physical therapy for treatment of their lower back pain and await results with the complementary care first. As I always tell my patients, I have no objection to their use of complementary medical treatments as long as it is safe and helps them feel better.

During my years of training to become a pharmacist, which was my profession prior to medicine, I learned that many of the drugs we rely on today were originally derived from plants and other botanicals. It therefore makes sense to me that many of the herbal treatments and other naturally occurring substances used in complementary care today very possibly have real therapeutic effects on the body. Now that I am using many of them, I have seen first-hand some amazing treatment successes that I never expected to see.

One example of this is the use of glucosamine for the treatment of early osteoarthritis. An improvement in cartilage growth has been suggested in arthritis sufferers using this dietary ingredient. Many of my osteoarthritis sufferers have incorporated this substance in their treatment regimens and have achieved some success in relieving their arthritis pain. Many have noted improved mobility not achieved with conventional anti-inflammatory medications.

Another substance, which I have recommended frequently, and has shown great promise as a therapeutic agent, is DHEA. With his permission, I would like to report the patient experience of a gentleman I will call "Gary," who is one of my patients with intractable chronic fatigue syndrome.

Gary is a very pleasant 52-year-old gentleman who came to me complaining of severe fatigue for over six months. The fatigue had come on gradually, but had gotten to the point where he no longer had the energy to do activities with his family, which certainly bothered him. He was, at times, falling asleep at work, and really didn't feel like doing many things he used to enjoy. He had been very healthy all his life and had no chronic medical conditions.

Gary's life at work was stable and his home life, for the most part, was not stressful. But, his wife lately had been complaining of his loss of libido. He was also complaining of intermittent headaches and joint pains, which was a new symptom over the past six months. He was worried that something terrible was wrong and wanted a thorough work-up with me. He had no recent illnesses and had no other symptoms except a sore throat three months ago.

Gary's physical examination was completely normal and he was minimally overweight. He did not appear depressed, nor did he have any other localizing exam findings.

My approach to fatigue is to rule out medical conditions that can make patients tired, in particular, diabetes mellitus, hypothyroidism and anemia. Infectious diseases should also be considered. Gary and I embarked on a thorough lab work-up including chemistries, complete blood count, thyroid tests, liver function tests, EKG, Epstein Barr viral studies and a DHEA level. His lab work returned normal except for his Epstein Barr viral studies, which showed an elevated IgG antibody level at 1:640, probably indicating a distant infectious mononucleosis infection which may still be active. Also, his DHEA level was 425 ng/dl, which is low. See Table 1 for a description of DHEA levels in men and women.

DHEA Blood Test (Free, Unbound)

UNIT OF MEASURE		PRIME PEAK	GOOD	DEFICIENT	WORRISOME
ng/dl	Men	700-1200	450-700	170-450	Less than 170
	Women	450-800	300-450	120-300	Less than 120
ng/ml	Men	7.00-12.0	4.5-7.0	1.7-4.5	Less than 1.7
	Women	4.5-8.0	3.0-4.5	1.2-3.0	Less than 1.2
mcg/dl	Men	0.7-1.20	0.45-0.7	0.17-0.45	Less than 0.17
	Women	0.45-0.8	0.30-0.45	0.12-0.30	Less than 0.12

Table 1.

We therefore had ruled out diabetes, anemia and hypothyroidism, and were left with a possible chronic active infection with infectious mononucleosis and a deficiency in his DHEA.

Gary and I talked about the diagnosis of chronic fatigue syndrome. I told him that he was meeting all diagnostic criteria for the disease since we had ruled out the above systemic diseases. I told him there were no good, reliable treatments for the disease and that the duration was also quite variable, depending on the individual. Gary decided that he would increase his aerobic exercise and eat more regularly, which is a good foundation to begin with treatment. We also talked about supplementing his DHEA level, since he was deficient and also because I had previous successes using DHEA for chronic fatigue syndrome.

Gary was interested but wanted to try conservative

therapy first. I agreed and told him to come back in one month for a follow-up visit. Gary came back in a month but he was still miserable and quite fatigued. At this point, we talked again about DHEA and he decided it was time to try it. We started DHEA at 50 mg each day. Two months later Gary finally came back.

I walked into the room and could tell immediately he was feeling better. He had a glow of elation on his face and looked well-rested and serene—a big change from before. He told me that over the past two months he had slowly become less fatigued, to the point now where he felt full of energy. He also stated that his libido improved and he attributed his improvement to DHEA.

I was very pleased because chronic fatigue syndrome is so very frustrating to treat. Gary continues to do well, and on his return trips to the clinic he is no longer fatigued and is on a maintenance dose of DHEA at 50 mg per day.

DHEA has been a very useful treatment option in my practice, not only for chronic fatigue syndrome, but I have also had success using it for arthritis sufferers, patients with Alzheimer's disease and chronic pain syndromes.

DHEA has been called the "Mother Hormone." It is naturally produced by the adrenal glands in the body and subsequently metabolized to a number of other hormones, including the sex hormones, estrogens and testosterone. Its inherent properties make it particularly useful for a variety of diseases.

Also, we know that as people age, their DHEA levels begin to fall, until by age 75 to 80, there is only minimal amounts of DHEA left in the bloodstream. Some researchers think this deficiency may actually be the cause of some diseases.

Although these case histories are anecdotal, they are true individual patient experiences and represent a small sampling of what I have seen evolve in my practice. These and other patient successes lay the foundation for the BoomerAge Model having credibility in today's health care environment. Eventually, valid studies will be done as the model evolves, but many have said, "Why do we need more scientific studies, when we know that these complementary therapies have been around for hundreds of years, are safe and help people feel better?"

I think as long as complementary care is integrated with conventional care, this argument makes sense. In a system using complementary health practices as its sole treatment modality, where acute life-threatening medical problems are being treated with complementary methods, we should demand to see accurate double-blind placebo controlled studies that demonstrate efficacy for the problem.

Both systems of health care provide a valuable service to patients and have done so for hundreds of years. Let us not throw out one system to spite the other. Rather let us find the benefits and shortcomings in each system, integrate them and provide patients with a wide variety of treatment options for their health.

This will require an open-minded spirit of cooperation between the conventional providers of care and the complementary practitioners. From a conventional point of view, my interactions with the complementary providers, particularly the Naturopathic physicians, reveal that they are just as empathetic about their patient's problems as I am. Their style of healing is different than mine, but nonetheless effective. Most Naturopathic physicians that I have talked to are more than willing to support an integrated health model and they are willing to teach and provide insight to their method of healing.

In addition, as you can see from the surveys that have been done, the public, primarily the Boomers, are asking for this integration. They want the option of complementary practices they have been used to. Consequently, the BoomerAge Model becomes a new model for health care delivery with conventional and complementary health care providers working together toward a common goal - making their patients feel better.

There is a lot of work to be done to make the model a reality, but with the support of the many interested physicians I have met and the support of complementary medical community and the Boomers, the model should evolve into a system we are all comfortable with.

Lastly, the dietary supplement industry must work with us to provide reliable products with strong scientific support for safety and efficacy. Also, I would like to see this industry expand its research into new metabolic analogs of naturally occurring substances. It is my belief that there are hundreds and perhaps thousands of useful compounds as yet undiscovered which possibly have some therapeutic benefit to the human body.

With this expanded research to discover new and useful therapeutic compounds, and with the BoomerAge Model to provide physician-guided use of these supplements, I see many opportunities for improving health care in this country. The next chapter presents an example of how the dietary supplement industry responded to consumer needs originating from something I call the DHEA Dilemma.

CHAPTER THREE

The DHEA Dilemma

The dietary supplement industry has never been more active than it is right now. Since Congress passed the DSHEA Act in 1994, many new dietary supplements have been introduced to the market. Many industry research departments are busy investigating new natural products and some companies have advanced to finding derivatives or metabolic analogs of natural substances to change the properties of the parent compound. This research could be very helpful to the medical community by eliminating known side effects and improving the potency of these natural products.

One example is a more recent dilemma concerning the use of a naturally-occurring dietary supplement called DHEA. DHEA has been shown to have many positive qualities, but it also converts into testosterone and estrogens in the body. In some patients, these hormones are useful in increasing libido etc., but not recommended for people at risk of breast, uterine, ovarian or prostate cancer or prostate problems. Let us now review DHEA, its science and beneficial uses, and then consider a new metabolic derivative of DHEA that is more potent and eliminates these unwanted side effects.

Background on DHEA

DHEA is an acronym for a naturally occurring hormone produced by the adrenal glands, which sit on top of each kidney. See Figure 3.

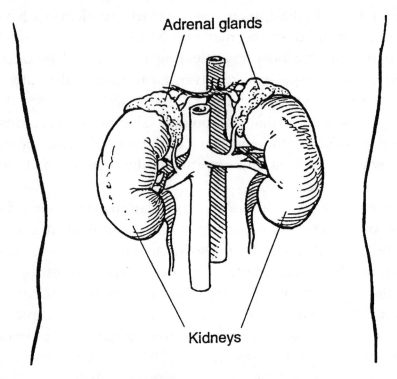

Human adrenal glands and kidneys.
Figure 3.

DHEA is known as dehydroepiandrosterone (de-hydro-epi-an-DROS-ter-own). DHEA is synthesized in the adrenal cortex from cholesterol via pregnenolone by the action of adrenocytochrome P450. Cytochrome P450 is an enzyme in the adrenal cortex that catalyzes this reaction. It is the most abundant adrenal steroid hormone in humans. The adrenal cortex also produces glucocorticoids (hydrocortisone or "cortisol") and mineralocorticoids (aldosterone). The term "corticosteroid" is often used to refer to any of the hormonal steroid substances obtained from the cortex of the adrenal gland and includes DHEA. Figure 4 shows the approximate daily production of adrenal hormones, including DHEA, by the adrenal cortex.

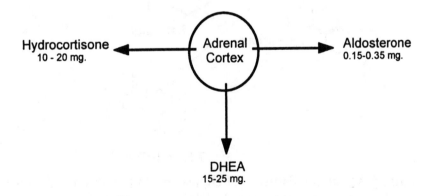

Daily production of adrenal hormones.
Vande Wiele et. al., 1960.
Figure 4.

See Figure 5 for the diagrammatic visualization of how DHEA is synthesized by the body and how it is metabolized to other adrenal hormones for use by the body.

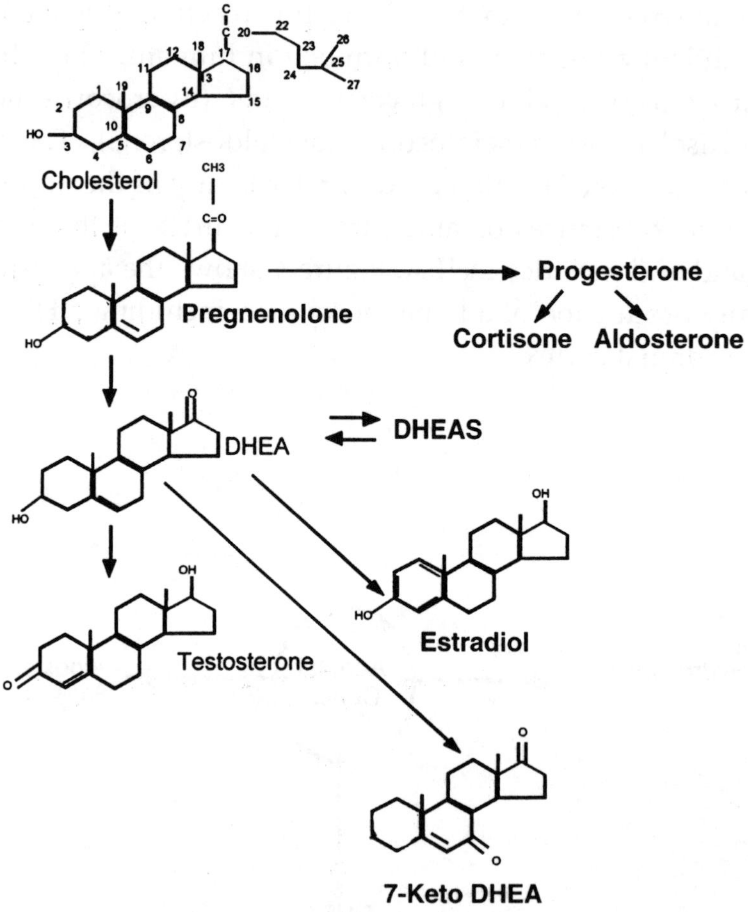

Figure 5. Metabolic Pathway of cholesterol in the adrenal glands illustrating its conversion to DHEA and other steroids.

Please note the numbering of the positions on the cholesterol ring structure, especially position 7, which will become important later when we talk about 7-Keto DHEA.

The DHEA Dilemma 43

Before being secreted into the plasma, most of the DHEA is sulfated at the number three position to form dehydroepiandrosterone sulfate (or DHEAS). This compound is the dominant steroid in the plasma in most mammals, including humans, where it exists at concentrations between one and six micrograms per milliliter.

The levels of DHEA increase through the second decade of life and then decrease with age. It is believed to have a protective effect until humans reproduce and then nature doesn't care any more. At age 80 years, one has about five percent as much DHEA as during the prime years[2]. Serum levels of DHEA in men are significantly higher then those of women at all ages from 20 to 69 years, probably reflecting testicular contribution to the serum pool.

This is illustrated in the study by Orentreich, et. al., in 1984 measuring DHEAS concentrations throughout adulthood, noting age changes and sex differences. They found that DHEAS concentrations peaked at age 20 to 24 years in men and at age 15 to 19 years in women. The mean values then decline steadily in both sexes. Levels in men were significantly higher than in women. This study did not find monthly, seasonal or annual variations in serum DHEA levels.

In contrast, serum levels of cortisol and other adrenal steroids remain relatively unchanged with aging. This results in a striking increase in the glucocorticoid/DHEA ratio as persons grow older[3]. This ratio is also a major biomarker for chronological age[4]. The physiological significance of the variation in DHEA plasma levels is unclear, albeit interesting. The fall in serum levels occurs as the incidence of diseases,

[2] Orenteich, et.al. 1984, Barrett-Connor, 1986, and Loria et.al., 1988.
[3] Svec, et. al., 1989.
[4] Migeon, et.al., 1957 and Orentreich, et. al., 1984.

such as cancer, heart disease, diabetes and obesity rise, suggesting that DHEA or DHEAS may be protective against their development.

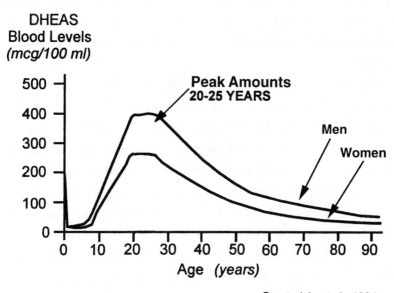

Figure 6.

As you can see from Figure 6, the levels of DHEA in men and women decline as they get older. The levels, in fact, reach their lowest levels at age 75, which currently happens to be the average age of death. Many researchers and writers on the subject have raised the question of a cause and effect relationship between DHEA levels and death. In other words, it may be that the decline in DHEA is not the effect of aging but a contributing cause of death.

If this assumption is actually true, keeping your DHEA levels at or near their younger age plateau could theoretically extend your life span and improve your quality of life by preventing chronic disease. A number of researchers working with DHEA have taken it themselves for years for exactly this objective.

The uses of commercially available DHEA are protean, and pharmaceutical grade DHEA is now widely available in the United States as a nutritional supplement. For instance, DHEA is used in conjunction with estrogens to reverse menopausal symptoms, and has also been used in the treatment of manic depression, schizophrenia and Alzheimer's disease. Lately, our research in the United States has shown DHEA to be a valuable treatment adjunct for a number of other disease states, all of which we will discuss later in this book.

Before we get into those uses, however, I think it would be valuable to introduce you to the human endocrine system. When I was in medical school, getting a clear understanding of why hormones exist and how they function in the body gave me tremendous insight into many bodily functions, and how hormone deficiencies resulted in disease states. That knowledge made the next step toward treatment of those diseases very easy. Although the system is complex, it can be broken down into language that is easy to grasp, and for our purposes, will make understanding DHEA as a hormone and as a treatment for certain diseases a logical progression.

Human Endocrine System

The human endocrine system is a masterful feat of design and functions as the body's regulatory mechanism. It has many parts but all interplay beautifully together to allow the body to function flawlessly. If the system is working, you feel well. If one or more of the parts are dysfunctional, you feel lousy.

First of all, the word endocrine is a descriptive term in reference to the body's various glands. If a gland is an endocrine gland, it releases a hormone into the bloodstream to affect a target organ. If a gland is an exocrine gland, that particular kind of gland releases the hormone directly to the target organ via separate ducts to affect a change.

One example of a gland that has both functions is the pancreas. The pancreas functions as an endocrine gland when it releases insulin into the bloodstream to lower blood sugar. It also acts as an exocrine gland when it releases amylase directly to the duodenum via ducts to help with the digestion of the food we eat.

The body has numerous important glands that make up the human endocrine system. They are the pituitary, adrenal, thyroid, parathyroid, pancreas, pineal, thymus, and men have testes and women have ovaries. Please see Figure 7 on the next page for a depiction of their locations in the male and female body.

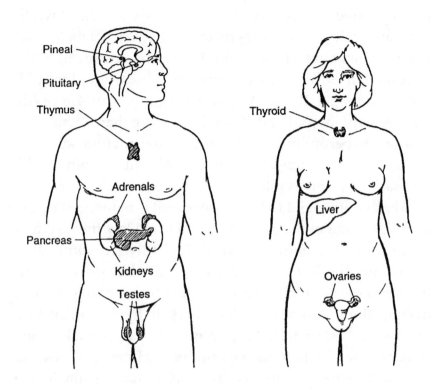

Male and female gland locations.
Figure 7.

Each gland has one or more hormones that are synthesized and secreted into the bloodstream or into ducts to affect their specific target organs. Most of the glands in the body function via an ingenious system we call a feedback loop. The amount of hormone that is secreted is regulated so that the correct amount is in the bloodstream at any given time. Let's look at an example of this to give you a better idea of how it works.

The thyroid gland, for instance, releases a hormone called levothyroxine or T4, which is the body's main thyroid hormone which basically regulates the body's metabolic rate. A normal amount of T4 in the human bloodstream, when measured in the laboratory, is anywhere from 4 to 12 mcg/dl (micrograms per 100 cc's). If you have less than 4 mcg/dl, you are hypothyroid and if you have more than 12 mcg/dl, you are hyperthyroid. So how does the thyroid know to secrete just the right amount of T4? This is where the feedback loop comes into play.

The amount of T4 in the bloodstream is monitored by the pituitary gland in the brain. If the T4 is too low the pituitary gland secretes a hormone called TSH (thyroid stimulating hormone). The TSH is released into the bloodstream and travels to the thyroid gland where it tells the thyroid to start making more T4 to raise the level back up to normal. Then as the T4 levels start to rise, it eventually travels back to the pituitary gland where the amount of TSH being released is gradually reduced until the T4 level is once again in the normal range. Ingenious, huh?

Therefore, in knowing each gland's hormone, stimulatory hormones and feedback loop, we can predict what diseases they may have by measuring the appropriate hormone or stimulatory hormone in the bloodstream. See Figure 8 for a visual description of what has just been described.

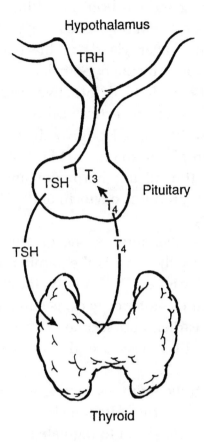

Thyroid feedback loop.
Figure 8.

One important point I would like to make at this juncture is that each gland may have one target organ it affects, or in some cases, several target tissues. This certainly predicts the importance of some glands versus others, as we consider a wide variety of endocrine diseases and their impact on the body.

The pituitary gland has been called the master gland, or as I have always called it Big Daddy. Its primary function is to control all the other glands in the body. Its secretory function is controlled by the hypothalamus in the brain.

The pituitary is divided into two areas: anterior and posterior. The anterior section produces TSH (thyroid stimulating hormone), GH (growth hormone), ACTH (adrenocorticotropin hormone), FSH (follicle stimulating hormone), LH (luteinizing hormone) and prolactin. The posterior section produces oxytocin and ADH (anti-diuretic hormone).

The pituitary, therefore, is one of our most important glands. ACTH, by the way, is the stimulating hormone for the adrenal cortex where DHEA is synthesized. The thyroid gland, located in the anterior neck, is stimulated by TSH, as we mentioned earlier, and secretes two thyroid hormones called T3 and T4. These are the body's main thyroid hormones.

The C-cells of the thyroid secrete calcitonin, which when released, decreases serum calcium. The C-cells work closely with the parathyroid gland to regulate calcium metabolism. Low levels of thyroid hormone result in a very common ailment called hypothyroidism. Hypothyroidism leaves patients with weakness, lethargy, weight gain and an inability to tolerate cold temperatures. With proper replacement therapy, all symptoms are controlled, but replacement is often life-long when started. The parathyroid glands are four small, pea-shaped glands on the backside of the thyroid. As mentioned, the parathyroid helps regulate calcium metabolism by secreting a hormone called PTH (parathyroid hormone).

The pancreas, as mentioned previously, has both exocrine and endocrine functions. Its endocrine functions occur within specialized cells called the Islets of Langerhans. The islets also contain a number of specialized cells called alpha cells, beta cells and delta cells. The beta cells are the most important of the three, and they have the daily duty of secreting insulin into the bloodstream for control of the body's glucose metabolism. Insulin, of course, regulates the body's blood sugar levels, and if deficient, a disease called diabetes mellitus results.

We have already talked about the adrenal glands, particularly the adrenal cortex, but it is also important to mention the adrenal medulla. The adrenal medulla secretes norepinephrine and epinephrine, which are neural transmitters for the sympathetic (fight or flight) nervous system. Adrenal insufficiency results in a disease called Addison's disease, which, by the way, afflicted President John F. Kennedy during his years in office. An excessive amount of corticosteroids results in a rather rare disease called Cushing's disease.

The gonads, which are ovaries in women and testes in men, each secrete their respective sex hormones, estrogens and testosterone. The ovaries, of course, also supply eggs for fertilization and the testes produce sperm for that process. FSH and LH from the pituitary gland act as stimulating hormones for the gonads and a very efficient feedback loop exists here as well.

The pineal gland in the brain is responsible for secreting melatonin and serotonin, which help to control the body's time clock, appetite and mood.

With that brief overview of the endocrine system, it will

now be a lot easier to understand the interactions of this system as it relates to DHEA and its metabolic analogs.

Getting back to DHEA now, I would like to discuss some of the more scientific aspects of DHEA to give us an idea of how DHEA reacts once it is inside the body when you take it in pill form.

Scientific Support

Pharmacokinetics of DHEA - Absorption

Little is known about the absorption of DHEA. Several studies, though, have been conducted showing DHEA taken by mouth is absorbed and metabolized in the body. For example, Leiter and his colleagues fed diabetic mice a diet containing 0.4 percent DHEA, which resulted in significant increases in serum DHEA (four to nine-fold increase).

This absorption was later confirmed by removing the glands in these mice that could possibly produce DHEA in the body on their own, thus falsifying their results from oral intake from DHEA. They removed the adrenal glands, testicles and ovaries and found that serum increases in DHEA after oral intake were exactly the same as those animals with all their organs remaining. We are, therefore, assured that when we take DHEA in tablet or capsule form, it will be absorbed into our own bloodstream and available to our end organs.

Upon administration of DHEA, some seems to remain in the body as DHEA, but a large amount becomes sulfated into

DHEAS. The DHEAS goes into a body pool where it is free to be distributed to the tissues.

The half-life of DHEA was determined in 1960 with research done by Vande Wiele. The half-life of a drug or substance is the time it takes for a serum concentration of a drug to fall by one-half of its original value. An example is if I injected substance X into your bloodstream and drew a level, that blood level would represent its peak concentration.

Let's say that your peak concentration was 100 micrograms/dl. Now we wait four hours and draw another blood level, and we find that it is 50 micrograms/dl. The half-life of substance X, therefore, would be four hours, since the blood level dropped by one-half of its original value.

One rule of thumb regarding the half-life is that it takes approximately five half-lives for a drug to nearly completely leave the body. In the case of substance X, it would take nearly 20 hours, or almost a whole day, for the drug to be metabolized and out of your system completely. This knowledge comes in handy when we are dealing with cases of poisoning or when we are changing medications in a patient. Vande Wiele found that the half-life of DHEA is a little over two hours.

Pharmacokinetics of DHEA - Distribution

DHEA originates largely from the adrenal glands, as we have already mentioned. This is known because DHEA increases in the urine with ACTH administration. Remember, ACTH is a stimulating hormone produced by the pituitary gland, which tells the adrenal glands to make more DHEA and other hormones. ACTH may be given artificially by injection into subjects, causing DHEA levels to increase.

Conversely, in conditions where ACTH is low, such as an ACTH secretion suppression syndrome, or when adrenal insufficiency (Addison's disease) is present, the levels of DHEA are low. By the way, there is some evidence that the testicles in males produce some DHEA, as proven in studies by dePeretti et. al., 1978.

DHEAS (the "S" signifies the sulfated form) is a metabolic conjugate (combination) formed in the liver from DHEA. There are also metabolic conjugates of other hormones as well, such as testosterone glucuronide and also conjugates of metabolites of DHEA, such as androsterone sulfate. This conjugation process takes places in the liver and is basically a parent compound being combined with a "salt" making it easier for them to circulate in the bloodstream.

The metabolic conjugates then circulate in the bloodstream, eventually reaching all organs and exerting either a hormonal or metabolic influence on the target tissue. As a further point of interest, almost all steroids produced in the body are conjugated with glucuronic or sulfuric acid before urinary excretion. Mean secretion rates, plasma concentrations and metabolic clearance rates are given for DHEA and DHEAS in Table 2.

	SECRETION RATE (MG/DAY[1])		PLAMA CONCENTRATION (G/100ML[1])		MCR (1 PLASMA/DAY[1])	
Steroid	Men	Women	Men	Women	Men	Women
DHEA	3.0	0.7	0.50	0.48	950	
DHEA-Sulphate	5.9	7.7	143	79	11	

[1]Mean secretion rates, plasma concentrations and metabolic clearance rates of DHEA and DHEAS. Data given are for healthy individuals aged 30-45 years. Secretion rate values are derived from plasma clearance studies. Gower and Honour, 1984.

Table 2.

Pharmacokinetics of DHEA - Metabolism

As already mentioned, in humans, DHEA produced by the adrenal glands is sulfated by an enzyme to DHEAS. More than 99 percent of the circulating DHEA is in the sulfate form. DHEAS circulates in the blood of humans at a much greater concentration than any other steroid hormone. Although the sulfated form is present in much larger quantities, it is thought that the active form of the hormone is the unsulfated form (free-DHEA)[5].

The conversion of DHEAS to DHEA is the first step in tissue specific metabolism to other steroid hormones. Therefore, the high level of circulating DHEAS provides a reservoir of substrate for the bio-synthesis of downstream steroid hormones, in other words, metabolites of DHEA.

When DHEA is given orally, it is sulfated to DHEAS in several tissues, including the intestine, liver, skin and possibly others. These two compounds are thought to be almost inter-convertible in most tissues of the body. The

[5] Schinazi et. al., 1989 and Lardy Personal Communication, 1997.

levels of DHEAS are probably determined, to a considerable extent, by rates of sulfation and desulfation in tissues[6].

In the human body, DHEA is converted to androstenediol and androstenetriol by an enzyme in the adrenal gland. This reaction, and others, probably convert DHEA to other metabolites as well. It is thought that this reaction is dependent and restricted by concentrations of DHEA and DHEAS in the circulation.

There is controversy about the action of DHEA. It is thought that about one-third DHEA is converted in the skin. It is speculated that after this conversion into metabolites, there may be spill-over into the blood to affect the immune system via an endocrine release into the circulation.

It is also speculated that the skin may interact directly with the immune system in its own way without the compounds going through the blood and acting like hormones. The mechanism of action is unknown at the present. No receptor for DHEA has yet been found[7].

It has also been found that human skin absorbs and metabolizes DHEA to testosterone. Recent studies have also indicated that DHEA is converted to androstenediol and androstenetriol in the skin[8]. Regelson and coworkers feel that this pathway is the one by which DHEA exerts its immunostimulatory affect, since androstenedione and androstenetrione act as regulators of immune system response in the body.

It therefore appears that DHEA is active in its "free" form and indirectly through many different metabolites produced in many different organs with the skin being most prominent. We are also getting some initial early clues to its uses including regulating the immune system.

[6] Roberts et. al., 1990
[7] Padgett, 1996.
[8] Faredin et. al., 1970 and Regelson et. al., 1990.

Pharmacokinetics of DHEA - Secretion

The normal corticosteroid secretion pattern is characterized by one in which peak corticosteroid concentrations occur prior to, or at the time of, awakening, and then decline over the remainder of the 24-hour period. Thus, in humans, peak concentrations are seen in the early morning hours and in nocturnal animals, the peak concentrations are seen in the early evening hours.

There are also superimposed episodic, relatively synchronous peaks of plasma corticosteroid concentrations throughout the day. The majority of these peaks occur in humans at the time of the circadian rise (3 a.m. to 9 a.m.) with other bursts seen most frequently in relation to mealtimes. There appear to be six to nine major secretory episodes per 24 hours. The normal serum, or plasma levels, of cortisol in humans are:

8 a.m.   5-25 micrograms/dl
8 p.m.   less than 10 micrograms/dl

Knowing these secretion patterns is very useful when adjusting oral corticosteroid medications, including DHEA. We would, therefore, dose these medications to match the body's own secreting rhythm. This puts the least strain on the pituitary and adrenal glands. You don't want to mess with Mother Nature, at least not very much anyway.

Plasma corticosteroid secreting concentrations are altered in a variety of human diseases. Examples include liver disease[9], Cushing's disease and advancing lung cancer[10], pituitary disease[11], acute or chronic diffuse CNS disease[12] and

[9] Tucci et. al., 1966.
[10] Sholiton et al., 1961.
[11] Krieger, 1973.
[12] Apfelbaum et. al., 1974.

depression[13]. Modern air travel (jet lag) also contributes to an alteration in corticosteroid secreting rhythm.

Early work investigating the variations in plasma levels of DHEA and androsterone was done by Migeon et. al., 1957, using 65 normal adult males and 31 normal adult females. Table 3 shows the day to day variations in plasma DHEA levels in five normal adult males as compared to their levels of corticosteroids.

Note that when DHEA levels are high, corticosteroid levels are low. Diurnal variations in plasma DHEA levels are shown in Table 4. There are also variations occurring in regard to the menstrual cycle in women, as illustrated in Table 5. Lastly, in post-menopausal women, DHEA levels were at or near zero. See next pages for Table 3, Table 4, Table 5, and Figure 9.

---

[13] Fullerton et. al., 1968.

Day-to-day Variation of Plasma DHEA and Corticosteroid
Levels in 5 Normal Adult Males. Migeon et. al., 1957

Subjects		Plasma DHEA (µg./100 ml.)			Plasma corticosteroids (µg./100 ml.)		
No & Name	Sex & Age	Sample 1	Sample 2	Sample 3	Sample 1	Sample 2	Sample 3
#9 P.H.	M 24	48.5	44.3	51.0	14.5	27.0	31.0
#11 C.P.	M 25	47.0	43.0	32.5	20.3	9.0	13.5
#19 P.B.	M 26	69.0	60.5	61.0	26.0	24.5	24.0
#20 M.R.	M 26	43.0	60.0	48.0	33.8	37.0	32.0
#28 M.H.	M 31	82.5	94.0	87.0	24.5	16.2	18.0

Table 3.

Diurnal Variation of Plasma DHEA and Corticosteroid
Levels in 13 Normal Adult Subjects (10 Men and 3 Women)
Migeon et.al., 1957

No. & Name	Sex & Age	Plasma DHEA (µg./100 ml.)										Plasma Corticosteroids (µg./100 ml.)							
		8 a.m.	9 a.m.	10 a.m.	12 noon	4 p.m.	10 p.m.	2 a.m.	4 a.m.	6 a.m.	8 a.m.	8 a.m.	9 a.m.	10 a.m.	12 noon	4 p.m.	10 p.m.	2 a.m.	4 a.m.
#47 P.	M 48	31.8					13.9	23.4	19.2		27.8	20.3					18.8	13.5	13.5
#19 P.B	M 26	69.0					53.5	56.0	57.0		70.0	26.0					15.5	13.0	19.3
#66 C.C.	F 29	31.2					26.4	21.0	9.6	33.0	30.6	19.0					16.8	12.0	7.4
#39 H.B.	M 40	38.5					30.1		28.0	43.7	32.5	30.0					19.6	25.0	22.5
#40 B.R.	M 40	36.0					29.4	31.9	31.9		38.4	23.0					19.3	12.2	10.8
#52 F.	M 54	55.0	54.5	36.2	28.8	35.5					46.5	27.6	20.4	16.3	14.5	8.0			
#38 L.	M 39	22.0	17.5	14.5	13.5	11.5					22.3	10.5	16.5	16.0	11.0	11.0			
#49 D.	M 51	15.2		5.0	10.4	10.0					21.0	7.5	8.3	5.0	7.1	6.0			
#44 B.E.	M 45	31.2	29.5	23.2	25.6	26.0					17.5	12.9	10.1	9.5	13.3				
#3 F.F.	M 22	36.5			30.5	28.2	25.8	24.0	29.2		33.3	23.8			23.4	22.0	20.4	17.4	20.5
#67 S.B.	F 23	65.5			60.0	72.0	65.5	33.8	65.0	61.0		21.0			23.0	32.0	29.5	22.7	16.6
#68 P.C.	F 23	36.2			32.2	24.2	20.6	14.5	36.0		34.0	13.0			10.3	11.2	10.0	8.9	13.1
#41 M.T.	M 41	23.7			28.5		26.0	35.0	24.2	27.5	31.0	10.7			13.2	8.9	8.5	3.5	4.5

Table 4.

Effect of the Menstrual Cycle on the Levels of Plasma DHEA and Corticosteroids
in 16 Normal Adult Females   Migeon et. al., 1957

| Subjects | | Plasma Levels DHEA (µg./100 ml.) | | | | | | | |
| No. & | Age | DHEA | | | | Corticosteroids | | | |
Name	(yrs.)	1*	2	3	4	1*	2	3	4
69 J.D.	25	45.5	56.5	33.0	—	29.5	36.5	17.0	—
70 P.W.	27	34.0	50.0	32.5	39.0	21.0	30.0	19.5	21.4
71 E.K.	24	38.0	50.0	29.5	—	25.5	25.6	9.7	—
72 A.S.	27	51.0	68.0	39.3	—	32.5	27.0	28.5	—
73 T.D.	29	19.8	18.2	14.3	16.4	10.0	3.3.	10.1	11.5
74 L.H.	25	45.0	58.5	54.0	45.0	19.1	15.6	13.9	16.3
75 M.F.	21	58.0	81.0	63.5	51.0	13.5	17.5	12.0	15.3
76 R.C.	26	59.5	50.0	48.0	—	37.0	26.2	23.0	—
77 S.R.	22	9.1	14.0	8.1	19.7	0	7.4	0	4.7
78 G.S.	24	34.0	32.6	22.0	36.5	48.5	38.0	22.5	40.0
79 L.F.	25	50.5	54.0	36.0	45.4	9.0	13.5	26.5	23.8
80 C.W.	23	52.0	32.6	—	45.0	24.5	19.3	17.9	37.8
81 A.B.	23	41.6	26.0	39.5	—	24.5	17.5	26.0	—
82 J.D.	24	78.0	53.0	68.0	—	25.0	32.5	22.6	—
83 P.B.	22	16.6	16.6	17.0	0	1.7	0	0	0
84 J.F.	25	64.0	—	50.4	—	25.0	38.0	21.6	—
Average±S.D.		43.5 ±17.5	44.1 ±19.0	37.0 ±16.9	33.2 ±16.4	21.5 ±12.3	21.7 ±8.2	17.0 ±8.3	18.9 ±13.1

*1=2 days after beginning of menstruation.
2=2 weeks after beginning of menstruation.
3=3 weeks after beginning of menstruation.
4=2 days after beginning of following menstruation.

Table 5.

Rosenfeld et al., 1975, conducted a 24-hour secretory study in a 42-year-old normal male, shown in Figure 9. DHEA concentrations were measured every 20 minutes over 24 hours. There were at least nine peak episodes in the secretory pattern of DHEA in this subject. In each instance, a corresponding peak of cortisol concentration was found at or near the DHEA maximum.

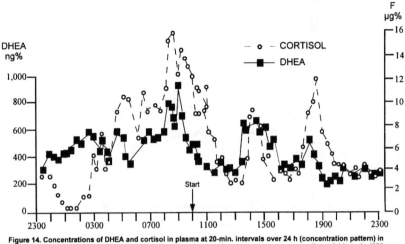

Figure 14. Concentrations of DHEA and cortisol in plasma at 20-min. intervals over 24 h (concentration pattern) in normal male (42 yr.)   Rosenfeld et. al., 1975

Figure 9.

Maximum secretory activity occurred between 5 a.m. and 10 a.m. with additional peak periods of activity between 1 p.m. and 3 p.m. and between 5 p.m. and 7 p.m. The mean 24-hour concentration of DHEA obtained as an arithmetic mean of the 72 samples taken over the 24-hour period was 512 ng/dl, with values ranging between 300 and 950 ng/dl. The half-life of endogenous plasma DHEA varied from 67 to 186 minutes. Figure 10 illustrates the DHEA half-life in the 42-year-old male subject.

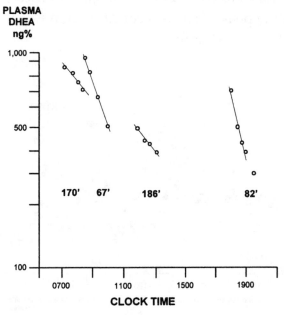

Half-lives of endrogenous DHEA during 4 periods where concentration is decreasing. Same subject as in Figure 10.   Rosenfeld et. al.,1975

Figure 10.

In a study by Sirinathsinghju and Mills (1985), plasma levels of DHEA, along with other adrenal androgens, were measured in eight normal women every two hours for ten hours. There were significant diurnal variations in the levels of DHEA, with the high levels in the morning and the low levels in the evening. Villette et. al. (1990), measured alterations in the secreting rhythms of the secretions of several hormones in HIV infected males. As compared with normal control subjects, the 24-hour mean concentrations were significantly higher for cortisol and lower for DHEA and DHEAS in all HIV infected patients.

During timed measurements of plasma hormone levels,

an altered secreting rhythm pattern of adrenal hormones was clearly indicated in HIV infected subjects. It was speculated that some stimulating substance, perhaps secreted by the infected immune cells, was causing these effects. This information will become very important to remember when we start talking about DHEA and its benefits in HIV infected patients, particularly in regard to immune system response.

Pharmacokinetics of DHEA - Excretion

The first to show that DHEA was excreted by humans in urine was Leiberman (1948). Since then, several others have determined the presence of DHEA in urine[14]. According to Gower and Honour (1984), most of the DHEA urine excretion occurs in the sulfate form, in amounts approximating 0.72 mg per day in men and 0.56 mg per day in women.

Vande Wiele et. al. (1963) determined the secretion into conversion and excretion rates of DHEA and DHEAS as illustrated in Figure 11.

[14] Gallagher, 1958; Lopea et.al, 1967 and Sonka, 1976.

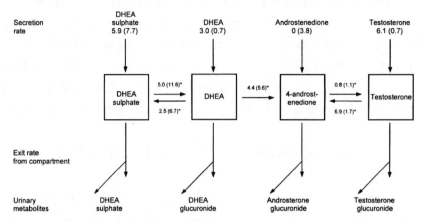

Secretion, interconversion and exit rates of DHEA sulphate, DHEA, 4-androstenedione and testosterone. All values are in mg. day of DHEA. The values given first are from a normal man; those in parentheses are from a normal woman. * Indicates interconversion rates. Vandewiele et. al., 1963.

Figure 11.

DHEAS, DHEA, androsterone and testosterone exit the body in the urine as DHEAS, DHEA glucuronide, and rosterone glucuronide and testosterone glucuronide, as illustrated.

Mechanism of Action

Steroids are thought to act by binding to specific receptors present in the cytosol (the liquid medium of the cell), or the nuclei (the brains of the cell), or both. Most steroidal compounds exert their effects by interacting directly with the glucocorticoid receptor, either at its agonist site (the direct receptor site) or at its antagonist site.

At present, DHEA's mechanism of action is unknown; there are many theories. DHEA may act directly on targeted cells and also indirectly through systematically buffering other steroids[15]. It is not known whether DHEA acts alone, as its metabolites, or as a combination. Whether there is a DHEA receptor site and where that site is located is in debate.

Several theories have been postulated. DHEA may bind directly to the glucocorticoid receptor and antagonize glucocorticoid actions. Shafogoj et. al. (1992), evaluated DHEA's ability to displace dexamethasone (a potent cortisol derivative) from cytosolic receptors in a rat and found it did not do so.

Another possible mechanism of action is that DHEA may directly modulate glucocorticoid receptors. Kalimi et. al (1990), found that giving DHEA to rats for five days (4 mg/100 grams body weight) reduced glucocorticoid receptors in the liver by 50 percent. It has not been determined whether this holds true in other target tissues.

In the lab, Kalimi, et al. (1990), discovered that rat liver cytosol exhibits high affinity and a specific binder for DHEA. The specific binding was highest in the liver, followed by the kidney and testes. It has yet to be determined if this binder

[15] Regelson, 1994

has any physiologic relevance that would identify it as a specific receptor.

Another possible mechanism of action as it relates to the immune system was investigated by McLachlin et al. (1996). They studied DHEA modulation of monocytes. Monocytes can be thought of as surveillance cells in the body. They are one of the first cells in the body to encounter foreign elements in an effort to destroy them. Monocytes act in two ways: the first is by binding to the foreign element and engulfing it; the second is by releasing specific "attack" mediators, including interleukin 1 (IL-1) and tumor necrosis factor (TNF).

The findings in this study concluded a positive action of . DHEA on the immune system. Data also indicated the presence of a DHEA receptor in monocytes. During serious illness, there are characteristic increases in serum cortisol concentrations and urinary cortisol excretion with a shift in steroid metabolism away from DHEA and DHEAS to that of the glucocorticoids instead. This holds true in immune response with glucocorticoids and DHEA being antagonistic toward each other.

In addition, the increased glucocorticoid concentrations directly affect the immune system in a negative way, injuring it and leaving the patient vulnerable to pathologic processes normally held in check by the adequately functioning immune system[16].

Studies show that DHEA can be used to up-regulate the host immune response to viral infections by increasing the number of antibody forming cells, by increasing the number of white blood cells associated with resistance to virus infection and by markedly reducing virus induced mortality.

Virus (antigen) has to be present in order to demonstrate DHEA's up-regulation of the body's immune response.

DHEA's action on the immune system is a very important discovery, as we will realize during our discussions of DHEA uses.

DHEA In Your Life

By now, it is quite clear that DHEA is a naturally occurring steroid, and actually, the most abundant of them all. DHEA is also available in a pharmaceutical grade tablet or capsule as a nutritional supplement that you can buy over the counter. For years now, researchers and the general public have taken supplemental DHEA every day to promote wellness or to treat disease states.

Certainly if you read the many books on the market today about DHEA, you will find DHEA promoted as a useful treatment for aging, improving libido, increasing energy, boosting the immune system, reducing body fat, building lean muscle mass and as a protection against major diseases. But how much of this is true? How much DHEA are the people taking and what are the side effects and long-term treatment complications?

For instance, since I began writing this book, I have become advised that many people around the country are taking DHEA in amounts approaching 1000 to 2000 mg per day to promote muscle mass. They report that the improvement in muscle mass is astounding, but at what price? There simply are not enough good clinical studies using DHEA in this manner to testify to its safety in higher doses.

With an open mind, I have reviewed the existing literature available for DHEA in the treatment of various diseases. Let us now take a look at what we know about DHEA and the treatment of diseases. What diseases and conditions can be cured and modified? What are the side effects of treatment? What are the doses and are those doses safe for long-term treatment? Along the way, I will try to include as much human clinical data as possible; however, some animal data will be presented as well, to illustrate some of the possible future uses of DHEA.

DHEA and DHEAS have had wide clinical experience. Both have been used in human clinical trials in treating menopausal symptoms, high cholesterol, arteriosclerotic heart disease, gout, cirrhosis, lupus and Alzheimer's disease, to name a few.

Heart Disease

Heart disease remains the leading cause of death in the United States, and is by far the most common complaint I encounter in my clinical practice. Since it is the leading cause of death, it gets a lot of attention in the medical and also the lay press. Everyone by now knows the common risk factors for heart disease, which include cigarette smoking, diabetes mellitus, high blood pressure, high cholesterol, male sex and a positive family history for heart disease. Modification of some of these risk factors is possible, and some, such as male sex and family history, are a little more difficult, if not impossible, to change or eliminate.

The medical literature has already proven that lowering your serum cholesterol will decrease your chances of having a coronary event. In addition, a study done by the Veteran's Administration some years ago proved that taking an aspirin each day will decrease your chances of having a heart attack by 50 percent.

We have also heard a lot about antioxidants lately, with Vitamin C and Vitamin E being good examples. Antioxidants may prevent coronary events by their action on cholesterol. When cholesterol oxidizes in the bloodstream, it has a greater affinity to "stick" to the inside of the arterial walls, which may in turn, result in a cholesterol plaque. Antioxidants prevent this oxidization process, thereby keeping our arteries open so that our heart muscle gets as much blood supply as possible.

So is there any way DHEA levels are linked to heart disease and would DHEA supplementation be of any benefit in the prevention of coronary disease? One important fact that we know from studies done by Mitchell (1994) and Barrett-Connor (1995) is that serum DHEAS levels are inversely related to premature heart attack in males, and that this association is independent of the effects of several known risk factors for premature heart attack.

In other words, these studies found that men who had premature coronary events had lower levels of DHEA than a control group. There was no association in women. Does it then follow that replacing DHEA in men who are deficient in it result in fewer heart attacks in these men? Unfortunately, the answer to this question is unknown, but probably should be studied in a larger, double blind cross-over study.

In my research on the subject so far, I have found no convincing data that DHEA lowers cholesterol or in any way has a favorable impact in blood lipids. What I have found, however, is some convincing evidence that DHEA may act as a "blood thinner" and through that mechanism prevent coronary events.

As you probably know, the most common cause of a myocardial infarction (heart attack) is a clot that has formed and is occluding a coronary artery. This stops blood flow to the heart muscle and part of the heart muscle dies, resulting in the infarction (dead tissue). We know that one of the first steps in clot formation is platelet aggregation. Platelets are small cells in your bloodstream that act to prevent leaking from small tears or other defects in your arteries. They essentially "plug" the holes. Aspirin prevents the platelets from sticking together, thereby making clot formation difficult.

In a study done at the Medical College of Virginia[17], five male volunteers were given 300 mg of DHEA three times daily for two weeks. They tested their platelet aggregation rates compared to a placebo group. They found that four out of five men on DHEA had prolonged platelet aggregation rates. Since we know that aspirin prevents 50 percent of coronary events through this same mechanism, one certainly could postulate that DHEA supplementation may result in similar outcomes.

Aging

As discussed earlier, we know that DHEA levels decline with age. In fact, after age 20, there is a progressive down slope in the blood levels to age 80, where they are probably five percent of their earlier values. One would wonder whether we could influence longevity by long-term supplementation with DHEA.

---

[17] Jesse, Loessner et. al.

Theoretically this idea makes sense and may well be true, but more studies need to be conducted primarily to rule out possible negative effects of long-term use. What particularly worries me are the possible long-term effects of DHEA's conversion into the sex steroids, testosterone and estrogens. Hormone responsive tumors, such as prostate cancer and breast cancer, may flourish in such an environment.

Menopause

In a random placebo controlled cross-over study by Mortola and Yen (1990), the pharmacological effects of DHEA were evaluated in six post-menopausal women, all 30 to 50 percent over ideal weight. The women were given four 400 mg doses of DHEA or placebo for 28 days (1600 mg per day). Refer to Table 6 for a summary of the results.

A prompt and dramatic increase in all serum androgen levels was observed after the first oral dose of DHEA. These effects were still obvious after 28 days on DHEA, peaking within two weeks and declining slightly thereafter. FSH and LH levels were unchanged. Placebo treatment did not alter any of these parameters. Serum cholesterol declined 11.3 percent within the first week of DHEA treatment.

This change was maintained throughout the 28 days, along with a 20 percent decline in HDL (high density lipoprotein, or good cholesterol). LDL (low density lipoprotein, or bad cholesterol) and VLDL (very low density lipoprotein) and total triglycerides showed a downward trend, but were not significantly lower during DHEA treatment as compared with placebo. Mean body weight did not change significantly; percent body fat was also unaltered. Dietary intake was similar in both treatments.

Physical measurements and laboratory characteristics
before and after 28 days of treatment with DHEA
and placebo in six postmenopausal women

	DHEA		Placebo	
	Day 0	Day 28	Day 0	Day 28
Wt. (kg)	80.8 ± 1.9	82.2 ± 1.9	81.4 ± 1.8	82.2 ± 1.7
	(75.0 - 87.2)	(77.7 - 87.7)	(75.0 - 85.0)	(76.4 - 85.9)
% IBW	140 ± 3	143 ± 3	142 ± 2	143 ± 3
	(130 - 150)	(134 - 155)	(134 - 150)	(135 - 155)
Weight index	11.4 ± 0.1	11.5 ± 0.1	11.6 ± 0.1	11.5 ± 0.1
	(11.4 -12.0)	(11.1 - 11.8)	(11.3 - 12.0)	(11.1 - 11.8)
% Body fat	47.3 ± 0.9	47.3 ± 0.7	47.5 ± 0.6	47.3 ± 0.6
	(45.7 - 51.2)	(45.7 - 50.1)	(45.9 - 49.3)	(45.9 - 49.5)
LH (IU/L)	118 ± 20	112 ± 11	107 ± 17	116 ± 19
	(76 - 141)	(71 - 183)	(75 - 156)	(81 - 172)
FSH (IU/L)	118 ± 12	119 ± 10	115 ± 13	113 ± 11
	(95 - 160)	(87 - 148)	(89 - 151)	(87 - 142)
Glucose (fasting, nmol/L)	4.2 ± 0.2	3.9 ± 0.3	4.2 ± 0.3	4.1 ± 0.2
	(3.8 - 4.9)	(2.8 - 4.4)	(3.3 - 4.9)	(4.0 - 4.6)
Insulin (pmol/L)	114 ± 32	118 ± 31	119 ± 35	112 ± 25
	(57 - 287)	(64 -238)	(57 - 202)	(79 - 281)
GbPD (IU/g hemoglobin)	8.9 ± 1.0	8.8 ± 0.7	9.1 ± 0.1	8.5 ± 0.4
	(8.5 - 9.7)	(7.9 - 9.8)	(8.9 - 9.7)	(7.0 - 10.0)

The range is given in parentheses. IBW, Ideal body weight.   Mortola and Yen, 19

Table 6.

A rise in serum DHEA and DHEAS between 60 and 180
minutes after DHEA administration suggests that rapid
sulfation of circulating DHEA occurred and reflects an
abundance of tissue steroid sulfatase in post-menopausal
women. No abnormalities in physical examination, liver
function tests (LFTs), complete blood counts or urinalysis
were seen. No appetite changes or sex drive changes were

reported, and no adverse consequences were noted. When administered in this manner, DHEA will raise the level of serum androgen (testosterone) in post-menopausal women. Unfortunately, the effect of DHEA on estrogens levels in these women was not monitored.

Osteoporosis

Osteoporosis, or a loss of bone mineral density in women is a common ailment I see in my clinical practice. Being an Internist, I see many geriatric men and women, and many of the elderly women I see have osteoporosis. Patients with osteoporosis are more prone to fractures, chronic pain and early arthritis. Physicians treat osteoporosis with estrogens supplementation and calcium replacement. Since DHEA is metabolized to estrogens, it would be theoretically useful for treating these patients.

Nowata et. al. (1995), tested bone mineral density and DHEAS levels in 120 post-menopausal women (51 to 99 years old) and found a direct correlation between DHEAS levels and bone mineral density. He found that women with higher DHEA levels had high bone mineral density (stronger bones). He also found osteoblasts, which are cells in our skeletal system involved in bone formation, are able to convert DHEA to estrogens. The study concluded that DHEA was important in maintaining bone mineral density in women after menopause.

What I tell my patients who want to take DHEA for osteoporosis is that I will have to decrease their dose of estrogens replacement based on the magnitude of their DHEA dose. I also tell them that taking DHEA will not only supply the estrogens they need, but also the testosterone. We have known for years that combined regimens of estrogens and testosterone not only relieves hot flashes and vaginal dryness but also the psychological symptoms such as mood changes.

Lupus

Systemic lupus erythematosus (SLE, lupus) has always been a fascinating disease state to me as a physician. It seems inconceivable that the body actually makes an antibody toward itself. The antibody is designed to destroy the nuclear material of cells disrupting their function. The exact cells attacked by the antibody vary from patient to patient, but very often affects vital organs such as brain and kidneys. Some clinical studies have been done with DHEA in treating patients with lupus. Here are a few examples with some encouraging results.

In a study giving ten females with SLE 200 mg doses of DHEA orally daily[18], DHEA showed promise as a new therapeutic agent for treatment of mild to moderate SLE. DHEA treatment for a three to six month period was well tolerated and with side effects, except for mild acneiform dermatitis (acne). Mild hirsutism was noted in two patients who were receiving Prednisone 10 to 20 mg per day, and some patients reported a decrease in menstrual flow with no changes in cycle. Mild acneiform dermatitis was also reported.

There were no adverse effects noted on physical examination or with laboratory evaluation. Eight of ten patients reported improvements in overall well being,

[18] Van Vollenhoven et.al., 1994

fatigue level and energy level. These patients elected to continue DHEA therapy for another three months. The study authors felt that their results were overall positive.

Van Vollenhoven et. al. (1995) completed another study using DHEA in SLE patients to further determine its benefit. This time, 28 women with SLE were treated with either 200 mg per day of DHEA or placebo, in addition to their usual medical regimen for a three month period. In this double blind phase, the women treated with DHEA showed improvement in each of four outcome measures (patients' self-assessment, physician assessment and a composite index of disease activity and Prednisone dose), while those on placebo worsened or remained stable.

After the initial three month study, 21 patients elected to receive open labeled DHEA treatment at 50 to 200 mg per day for three months. Those who previously had received placebo exhibited changes in their conditions similar to those who initially received DHEA. Again, mild acne was a frequently noted side effect (57 percent of patients). Other side effects, such as weight gain and abnormal menses were noted with similar frequency between the two groups. No adverse biochemical effects were noted. The study authors encouraged further studies of DHEA in the treatment of SLE.

Indeed, there are ongoing studies right now, evaluating DHEA and its benefits for SLE patients. Based on the above data to this point, DHEA may prove to be a valuable adjunctive treatment for SLE, a disease for which there is no cure.

Multiple Sclerosis

Multiple sclerosis (MS) is a disease of the central nervous system of currently unknown etiology. MS is exhibited pathologically by demyelination (loss of the nerve's protective myelin sheath), of white matter associated with mononuclear cell infiltrate consisting predominantly of T-cells and macrophages. This demyelination process is believed to be triggered by an infection, either viral or bacterial, which may result in aberrant immune reactions. There may be abnormal T-cell mediated auto-immune processes, as well as humoral immune abnormalities. As a result, plaque formation occurs and nerve conduction is impaired, leading to the disability seen in MS, such as numbness, loss of strength, double vision, etc.

Because of the positive roles demonstrated for DHEA in immune regulation (discussed later in this chapter), DHEA was hypothesized as potentially useful in treating MS[19]. DHEA was given at either 90 mg per day or 180 mg per day to chronic MS patients (nine females, 12 males). At the 90 mg per day dosing level, blood DHEA was elevated to normal or super-normal levels. Serum levels of DHEAS were also increased.

Improvements in some aspects of daily living were reported, such as improved mood, motor function, sexuality and energy level. On cessation of DHEA administration, these improvements gradually disappeared. It is unclear from this study whether DHEA administration resulted in any immuno-regulation of the multiple sclerosis in these patients, or whether the improved mood and energy levels were positive side effects of DHEA therapy. Clearly, further clinical studies are needed to investigate multiple sclerosis and DHEA.

[19] Roberts et. al., 1990.

Libido

There are no scientific human studies showing an improvement in sex drive. However, during my research for this book, I found hundreds of accounts from actual users of DHEA who reported improvement in libido, and this included both men and women. The improvements in libido cannot be proven positively and further studies may help with the answer to this question.

Sleep

DHEA has some affect on human sleep that should be mentioned for those persons thinking of taking it for other uses.

Friess in 1995 performed a study where 500 mg of DHEA was given to ten healthy men. In those men, a significant increase in REM sleep was noted. REM is an acronym for rapid eye movement sleep, or dream sleep. No other change in sleep pattern was found in these volunteers.

Therefore, in my practice, I cautioned my patients that they may have more dreams while they sleep if they are taking DHEA.

Diabetes Mellitus

Remember earlier when we talked about the endocrine system, and in particular, the pancreas. The beta cells of the endocrine pancreas secrete insulin. Insulin is responsible for transporting glucose into our cells for energy. A deficiency or resistance to insulin in our bodies results in a disease called diabetes mellitus.

A very common form of diabetes mellitus is called Type II diabetes. Very often Type II diabetes mellitus results because of a resistance to insulin, which develops as we get older. Obesity is also a cause of insulin resistance, and in patients prone to the disease, may result in the onset of diabetes.

In an interesting study done by Bates in 1995, DHEA was used to investigate insulin sensitivity. Fifteen post-menopausal women with an average age of 62 years were given 50 mg of DHEA over three weeks. This study showed an amazing increase in insulin sensitivity in these women. Their conclusions were that DHEA supplementation in post-menopausal women may decrease age related increases in insulin resistance.

This stimulating study certainly raises a number of questions, such as, would the same results be applicable to men? Would DHEA replacement in patients genetically predisposed to diabetes mellitus prevent or delay its onset? Would the same results be present in younger patients? I would love to see some long-term human studies on a larger focus population to study this theory further. I believe it may reveal some very valuable conclusions

Cancer

Most everyone would like to find a "cure" for cancer. It is certainly high on my wish list, having had countless patients die well before their time from a variety of different cancers. It is the second leading cause of death in the United States, behind cardiovascular disease. Lung cancer remains the most common malignancy in men and women, probably due to cigarette smoking. When I was in medical school breast cancer was the most common malignancy found in women; but that was soon overtaken by lung cancer, due to more women in the United States taking up smoking at that time.

It has been frustrating in my years as a physician to watch researchers working hard to find a cure for cancer only to be stifled by the myriad of pathways the carcinogen has in the body to cause a malignancy. The possibilities are endless and the cures, therefore, hard to find.

We know that genetics, smoking, sun exposure and diet probably have some role in the genesis and progression of cancers. What about adrenal steroids, and in particular, DHEA?

Unfortunately, since cancers take years to develop into serious malignancies, long-term human studies need to be done to prove the efficacy of anti-cancer agents. No long-term studies in humans have been done with DHEA. Many series of animal studies have been done primarily in rodents with variable results using DHEA as a tumor growth inhibitor.

Some studies actually show promising results using DHEA to inhibit the development of liver tumors in rats and breast cancer in mice. When you are talking about a disease as serious as cancer, that takes years to develop, we cannot rely on animal data to support treatment claims. Perhaps someday there eventually will be enough stimulus to study DHEA and its derivatives in the cancer arena, but for now, the effective DHEA administration in cancer prevention or treatment is inconclusive.

Claudication

One of the first studies conducted on DHEA in humans was in 1959 by Cask. He took six arteriosclerotic patients suffering from intermittent claudication (leg cramps upon walking due to poor circulation) and absent pulses in their feet. They were treated with 40 to 50 mg per day of DHEA for a period of one year. The results showed a definite symptomatic improvement in all patients. One hundred percent of the patients reported an improvement in their claudication. Also noted was a drop in serum total cholesterol from 416 mg/dl to 264 mg/dl after six weeks of treatment in one of the patients.

High Cholesterol

DHEAS was administered orally in doses of 20 to 80 mg daily to 13 subjects with high cholesterol to investigate effects on plasma lipids[20]. The treatment duration ranged from three to 42 weeks with some subjects receiving 80 mg doses of DHEA for as long as 42 weeks. No side effects were detected in any of the treatment groups. Patients did not observe any changes in general or psychological condition. No effects on routine hematological (blood cells) or by chemical tests were noted. DHEA had no effect on plasma lipid levels.

Immune System Function

Perfectly silent and unknown to us on a daily basis, our immune system is busy fighting off disease and foreign cells

[20] Adlercreutz et.al., 1972.

in our systems. The immune system is certainly complex and involves a well-coordinated system of cells and chemical mediators. The purpose of the system is to seek out and destroy any foreign bacteria, virus, disease cells, poisons or any kind of invader into our bodies. Not everything about the immune system is understood. What we know about it can be described briefly as follows.

The skin, of course, is our first line of defense, and if intact, will block a portal of entry to many foreign invaders. If a foreign substance manages to penetrate the skin barrier and enter our bodies, the next line of defense are our white blood cells.

There are many varieties of white blood cells in our bloodstream, but the polymorphonuclear cells (PMNs) and the lymphocytes are the ones we think of most often. Eosinophils and basophils are also a type of white blood cell involved in fighting infections (see Figure 12). The PMNs are actively involved in fighting bacterial infections, and their numbers increase and decrease with the presence of bacterial disease.

So, when your doctor tells you that your white count is elevated, he/she is usually referring to your PMN percentage, and telling you this should make you think primarily about a bacterial infection in your body, which is making you sick. For purposes of further discussion, let's focus our attention now on the lymphocytes. They are made in the bone marrow and there are two types: B-cells and T-cells. Since the terms will become important later, let us take a moment to define the players in this well-orchestrated game.

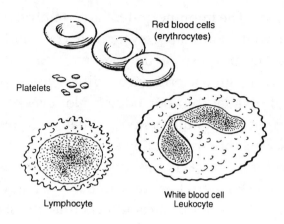

Human blood cells.
Figure 12.

T-Cells. A type of lymphocyte made in the bone marrow whose role is to fight against viruses, parasites and some cancers. There are two important types of T-cells: T-helper cells (CD4 cells) and T-suppresser cells (CD8 cells). The thymus, which is a gland in the upper chest, converts lymphocytes to T-cells, hence the name. The T-helper (CD4 cells) usually spend their time on searching missions throughout the body, looking for any foreign invaders. Once localized the T-helper cells will signal the T-suppresser cells to destroy the enemy or any signal the B-cells to produce antibodies against the foreign material.

B-Cells. Another type of lymphocyte made in the bone marrow, which, when mature, have the ability to make antibodies. They are found in the bloodstream along with the T-cells, monocytes and macrophages. Once an antibody is formed to a foreign substance the antibody attaches to it and neutralizes it.

NK Cells. Natural killer cells. Another type of white blood cell which acts as an efficient killer of cancer cells and some viruses. DHEA has been shown to increase numbers of NK cells in post-menopausal women.

Monocyte. A white blood cell found in the spleen, bone marrow and lymph nodes. Monocytes have a definite DHEA receptor on their cell surface. Monocytes function as a type of messenger releasing chemical mediators into the bloodstream activating a destructive cascade of events, which is focused on foreign invaders in our bodies.

Macrophages. Huge immune cells that kill foreign invaders by engulfing them. Macrophages respond to signals sent by B-cells and T-cells. They travel in the bloodstream or live in the spleen, liver or bone marrow.

Cytokines. These are very interesting proteins secreted by T-cells and Macrophages that help with cell destruction. Examples include interferon and interleukins.

Interferon. A type of cytokine released by lymphocytes to fight infections, particularly viral and some forms of cancer.

Interleukin. A protein similar to interferon secreted by T-cells to fight infections. Their purpose is to hunt down and attack foreign invaders. There are many different types of interleukins, and each has a different function. For example: IL-2 functions to signal other interleukins and interferon to activate the production of T-cells and B-cells in an effort to fight infections or cancers*.

Please see the glossary in the back for descriptions of other elements in the immune system.

There are many animal studies using DHEA showing some fascinating immune system up-regulation during

---

* Interleukin-1 (IL-1), Interleukin-2 (IL-2). Interleukin-3 (IL-3), etc.

infections. These results may or may not be applicable to humans.

Yen, in a study published in 1995, gave DHEA in doses of 50 mg per day to nine healthy, elderly men. Treatment with DHEA resulted in a definite increase in natural killer cells, increasing the numbers of NK cells in a person's body may certainly enhance the ability to ward off disease or other foreign invaders.

McLauchlan et. al. (1996) investigated DHEA modulation of monocyte cytotoxicity in monocyte cells. Monocytes, remember, can be thought of as surveillance cells. They are one of the first cells in the body to encounter foreign elements. Monocytes act in two ways: 1) directly, by binding to and engulfing target cells, mediated by specific receptors; and 2) indirectly, by releasing reactive oxygen/nitrogen intermediates and cytokines such as IL-1 and tumor necrosis factor (TNF). Their findings included a positive action of DHEA on the immune system. Data also indicated the presence of a DHEA receptor on the monocyte cell membrane.

Having a healthy immune system will not only help you feel better, you will be less prone to disease. Since a number of studies have shown that your immune system becomes more sluggish as you get older, taking DHEA in an effort to up-regulate your immune responsiveness makes a lot of sense, and certainly could allow you to live longer.

AIDS

AIDS (acquired immunodeficiency disease syndrome) is a disease characterized by the loss of cell mediated immunity and the development of frequent and eventually fatal opportunistic infections. The human immunodeficiency virus (HIV) is the etiologic agent of the acquired immunodeficiency syndrome (AIDS). Infection with HIV results in a profound immunosuppression due to the selective depletion of a subset of white blood cells known as Helper T-lymphocytes that express the receptor for the virus (the CD-4 molecule, also known as a T-4 cell).

Another major subset of T-cells express the CD-8 molecule on their surfaces (such cells are known as T-8 cells). These are classified as suppresser cells. The normal T-4/T-8 ratio is 1.5:1 to 2.0:1. In AIDS patients, this ratio is inverted due to a decrease in the absolute numbers of T-4 cells with normal numbers of T-8 cells usually being preserved.

The T-4 cells specifically recognize and proliferate in response to antigens that they encounter in the body, releasing proteins called lymphokines that regulate other immune system cells. The B-lymphocyte cells, upon signals from T-cells, recognize antigens and secrete specific antibodies to neutralize or eliminate antigenic bacteria and viruses traveling through body fluids. The T-4 cells also signal the T-8 cells to kill other cells infected with intracellular pathogens. These T-4 cells also modulate the activities of immune system cells, known as natural killer cells, and macrophages, which are involved in the response to infection and perhaps to incipient malignancies.

Early in HIV infection, the virus attaches via its envelope glycoprotein to the CD-4 molecule, a receptor on the surface of susceptible T-4 cells. The CD-4 molecule seems to bind the HIV virus, allowing infection and subsequent viral replication, as well as the cytopathic consequences of viral infection.

The immune deficiency of AIDS clearly demonstrates the importance of T-4 lymphocytes. The ability of AIDS patients to mount antibody reactions to new antigens is severely compromised due to fewer and less functional T-4 cells.

Monocytes serve as reservoirs for HIV and are relatively refractory to its cytopathic effects. A variety of inductive signals can convert HIV from a latent to a chronic active form in the human body. There is increasing evidence that macrophage/monocyte infection is a viral factor in the persistence and progression of HIV infection in initiating the cell damage that occurs in AIDS and in triggering the collapse of the immune system, as evidenced by eventual profound depletion of T-4 lymphocytes. The immunosuppression leaves the body open to various opportunistic infections and neoplasms.

The progression of HIV can be characterized by complex alterations in the production of adrenal steroids. The changes in steroid hormone concentrations during the development of HIV infection may have important implications for the immune response of patients. There is a relationship between cortisol levels and AIDS. Cortisol levels are increased in both the early and late stages of HIV infection—DHEA levels are decreased[21]. Even small changes in cortisol levels, such as those observed in the normal circadian rhythm can affect immune reactions[22]. The severity of this altered major hormonal system is predicted for progression to AIDS[23].

Plasma DHEAS levels were measured by Merrill et. al. (1989) in an aged matched blind study, as illustrated in Table 7.

[21] DePrato 1986; Membreno et.al., 1987; Christeff et.al., 1988 and 1992; Merril et. al., 1989.
[22] Herrscher et. al., 1992
[23] Jacobson et. al., 1991 and Mulder et. al., 1992

Human Plasma DHEAS Levels Compared with HIV Status

Condition of Individuals	Number Studied	Assay Results in μmol/L	P values
HIV negative	8	8.0 ± 2.4	
HIV positive apparently well	9	5.8 ± 1.7	P < 0.05
HIV positive with AIDS	10	3.9 ± 2.3	P < 0.001
Intra-assay coefficient of variation = 4.1% Inter-assay coefficient of variation = 12.2%			

Merril et. al., 1990

Table 7.

Eight healthy persons who were HIV positive had lower DHEA levels than nine HIV negative controls. Ten active AIDS patients had still lower values.

In a study done by Villette et. al (1990), HIV patients exhibited higher mean plasma cortisol levels and lower DHEA, DHEAS, and ACTH levels than controls. Analysis of the circadian rhythms of plasma hormone levels clearly indicated an altered adrenal hormonal state in HIV infected males, even during the asymptomatic period of infection.

These researchers speculated that increased cortisol secretion resulting from circadian varying stimulation of the adrenal cortex by something other than pituitary ACTH was the primary hormonal defect in HIV patients. This is certainly a thought-provoking study, leading one to speculate that HIV infected individuals somehow stimulate their adrenal cortices to secrete more cortisol at the expense of DHEA, and it is this progressive worsening of the cortisol/DHEA ratio that may eventually result in AIDS progression.

Jacobsen et. al. (1997) studied a group of 108 HIV positive men to determine the relationship between endogenous serum DHEA and DHEAS concentrations and HIV disease progression. Clinical and laboratory data were obtained at regular intervals over an extended time period. Over three and one-half years, it was concluded that serum DHEA levels below normal were predictive for progression of AIDS. This association persisted even after adjusting for hematocrit (red blood cell volume) and CD-4 lymphocyte counts, which are known to predict HIV disease progression, and age (DHEA declines with age, and age has been linked to HIV disease progression).

The association was significant only for individuals with CD-4 counts of 200 to 499; those with lower counts did not exhibit an association. This suggests that DHEA may be a relatively late stage marker and thus largely unrelated to disease progression in less immunosuppressed individuals.

Serum DHEA levels were found by Mulder et. al. (1992) to be lowest in AIDS patients, followed by HIV positive asymptomatic patients and lastly, by HIV negative controls. They concluded that a DHEA level of less than 7 nnol/l was an independent predictor for disease progression in HIV infected men.

In another study, Chatterton et. al. (1996) obtained blood samples from 16 HIV infected men with hemophilia and compared them to control samples from men without hemophilia or HIV infection. Before HIV infection, hemophiliacs had significantly lower plasma DHEA levels than controls. After infection, three of nine subjects studied serially for 11 years had little or no change in plasma DHEAS levels, or CD-4 cell counts.

In four men who developed AIDS, progressive decreases in DHEAS tended to precede falls in CD-4 cell counts. DHEAS plasma levels also decreased greatly in two other subjects who had other severe illnesses. None of the decreases in DHEAS levels were associated with decreased concentrations of plasma cortisol. These researchers concluded that plasma DHEAS is an indicator of general health, rather than a specific indicator for HIV progression.

Markham et. al. (1986) reported that the ability of HIV to infect normal human blood lymphocytes was greatly enhanced by supplementing the culture medium with corticosteroids.

It is believed that the AIDS virus induces this relative cortisol excess syndrome, but the mechanism of action is not known. Speculations include liver damage affecting the metabolism of cortisol and/or its antagonists, a central nervous system lesion affecting stress hormone integration, viral colonization of autonomic ganglia affecting endocrine glands, or another mechanism[24].

DePrato and his group proposed that a rational therapy of AIDS should involve:

1. Identification and removal/avoidance of stressors conducive to AIDS virus colonization.
2. Antiviral therapy.
3. Vigorous nutrient/energy repletion.
4. Anti-cortisol therapy with DHEA mentioned as a candidate.

DHEA-induced anticortisol therapy for HIV infected patients provides the hypothesis, then, for future human

[24] DePrato, 1986.

clinical trials using DHEA in its present form, or one of its derivatives, which would probably be safer for patients using long-term treatment.

Let me mention a couple more interesting studies to provoke your thought patterns in a different direction. It appears that there is a shift from Type-1 to Type-2 cytokine production during the progression of AIDS[25]. To explain further, HIV infection is associated with a progressive reduction in the Type-1 cytokines, interleukin-2 (IL-2) and interleukin-12 (IL-12), which both stimulate cell mediated immunity, and an increase in Type-2 cytokines, which are IL-4, IL-6 and IL-10. Type-2 cytokines stimulate humoral or antibody mediated immunity.

Because IL-12 and interferon gamma (IFN-gamma) are the main growth factors for Th-1 cells and IL-4 is the main growth factor for Th-2 cells, the normal homeostasis of the immune response is such that Type-1 cytokines tend to promote their own secretion and suppress the production of Type-2 cytokines, and vice versa. This phenomenon is reinforced by observations that IFN-gamma suppresses Th-2 cells and IL-4 and IL-10 suppress Th-1 cells. Which events initially destroy the equilibrium of the immune system, inducing a Type-1 to Type-2 shift is not totally clear.

Clerici et. al. (1994) suggested that the progressive shift from Type-1 to Type-2 cytokine production is partly provoked by the increased cortisol and decreased DHEA levels in HIV infection, leading to programmed cell deaths seen in AIDS. They speculate that by controlling the cortisol/DHEA ratio, the over-production of Type-2 cytokines might be reduced and the secretions of Type-1 cytokines increased, reducing programmed cell death and

[25] Clerici and Schearer, 1993.

interferon with viral replication in HIV infected cells. They suggested that this model could easily be tested in HIV positive patients.

The development of non-nucleotides (non-AZT type compounds) such as DHEA is important since the mechanism of action is different. This may make them suitable against potentially drug-resistant HIV variants or as alternative compounds to use alone or in combination with other drugs. Because DHEA is available orally, is relatively nontoxic and has a broad biological function, it may be a good alternative drug choice for HIV and AIDS. In addition, DHEA derivatives may be even more suitable due to their favorable side effect profiles in patients taking it for long-term use for control of this disease. In fact, later in the book we will see studies that bear this out using a new derivative called 7-Keto DHEA.

DHEA Dosing and Side Effects

Most of my concerns about DHEA focus on excessive, (exceeding 50mg daily) and uninformed or irresponsible use of DHEA. In order to achieve therapeutic benefit from DHEA, sometimes large doses are required over a long period of time. This however, can contribute to increased levels of the sex steroids testosterone and estrogens.

In my own clinical practice I use DHEA for a number of different diseases and complaints. Most of the time, I am striving to replace DHEA to its youthful levels, and therefore, a lot of my patients have serum DHEA levels done prior to administration.

Some of my patients come in asking for a DHEA level and

want to follow it as we treat them with DHEA supplements. I don't think pre-administration levels are universally indicated, but they certainly are interesting and revealing, and probably give me an extra clue to the etiology of a difficult medical problem.

DHEA is available over the counter as a nutritional supplement and usually comes in dosages of 10, 25 and 50 mg. The starting doses are variable, but as is the case with any new medication, starting with a low dose and working upward is always recommended. I usually start my patients out with 10 mg per day and work up to an average daily dose of approximately 25 to 50 mg per day.

Since DHEA is a steroid, and since most steroids follow circadian rhythms of secretion, I suggest that DHEA be given in the morning. After taking a dose of DHEA absorption is rapid, and usually in your bloodstream at about 60 minutes after ingestion. I usually make dosage increases every two weeks to give the body time to adjust to the dose and also to give the patient time to monitor its direct effects and its side effects.

Since DHEA is a fat soluble compound, it is better absorbed with a meal. Also, remember that DHEA is a potent hormone in the body and is metabolized to other active derivatives as well. Consulting with your health care provider before starting DHEA is definitely recommended.

Daily doses of DHEA should not exceed 50mg. Higher levels of DHEA supplements are not without their risks, and just because they are nutritional supplements doesn't mean they are innocuous. Here are a few of the potential high dosage side effects that contribute to the DHEA Dilemma.

Hirsuitism (hair growth) has been observed in females treated with DHEA. Lardy et. al. (1995) advises against using DHEA for extended periods in women because of an increase in male sex hormones. In a study by Yen (1990), 1600 mg per day of DHEA was given for 28 days, and there were rapid increases in serum androgen concentrations in six post-menopausal women.

These increased levels were maintained throughout the 28-day study, except for a slight decline at the end of four weeks. Adverse consequences of the increased androgens were not reported by the subjects, with the exception of one woman who had reported an increase in facial hair growth.

DHEA can act as a weight loss agent or an anti-weight gain agent, especially in animals, without changing food intake, in most cases[26]. In humans, body fat decreases have been observed in some studies[27], but not in others[28].

DHEA should not be taken by men with prostate enlargement due to its androgenic effects. One could also speculate that prostate cancer, since it is testosterone driven, may be made worse by DHEA. Women should also be aware of DHEA's estrogenic metabolites, possibly exacerbating breast cancer.

Other inconsistently occurring side effects of DHEA usually at high dosages have been reported in animal and human studies, including mild headache, insomnia, nausea, fatigue, skin rash, diarrhea, increased nasal congestion, vomiting and elevated plasma testosterone levels in rats and mice[29].

Several positive side effects of DHEA treatment have also been reported, including improved physical and psychological well being[30], and increased energy level[31].

[26] Cleary, 1983.
[27] Nestler, 1988.
[28] Mortola, 1987.
[29] Knudsen et. al., 1975; Regelson et. al., 1988; Schwartz et. al., 1988; and Loria et. al., 1989

[30] Roberts et. al., 1990 and Morales et. al., 1994.
[31] Roberts et. al., 1990 and Von Vollenhoven et. al., 1994.

Conclusions

It should now be clear that DHEA is a naturally occurring substance in the body and a plentiful one at that. It has areas of usefulness as a dietary supplement, but at high dosages (above 50mg daily) may have undesirable side effects.

The dietary supplement industry has responded to this DHEA dilemma by introducing 7-Keto DHEA as an alternative and more potent metabolic derivative. In an ideal world, this is exactly the way I would expect an industry to respond to a problem. The dietary supplement industry as a whole needs to continue to accelerate its research and develop more efficacious supplements for the medical community.

CHAPTER FOUR

7-Keto DHEA:
A Scientific Solution

7-Keto DHEA was developed as a natural extension of DHEA to enhance its benefits and eliminate side effects when taken at high dosages. In addition to the efficacy studies described in this book, 7-Keto DHEA will likely provide many of the benefits attributed to DHEA that are not associated with the production of sex steroids. For all of the reasons people have taken DHEA, 7-Keto DHEA will provide a more potent alternative.

Derivative Research

During my career as a pharmacist and physician, I have seen a number of drugs come and go. Some have withstood the test of time, like aspirin, Lanoxin and Inderal, to name a few. These favorite compounds are very useful because they have reproducible therapeutic effects and very few side effects and are therefore well tolerated.

The compounds which have been lost over the years were drugs that did not deliver a reliable treatment response, are dangerous in regard to their side effects, or cause actions on the body. There have also been a large number of useful drugs that have disappeared because they were replaced by derivatives. Seldane, for example, was an effective allergy medicine that was linked to heart problems. It was then replaced by a more potent drug called Allegra that does not have the risky side effects.

These derivatives are usually structural analogs of the same drug, and because of the chemical changes to the molecule, they either provided a better, more reliable therapeutic response, or had less side effects and were better tolerated than the initial agent.

Pharmaceutical companies have been creating derivatives of their own drugs for years, always striving for a better compound. I am not aware of any derivative of a nutritional supplement until now. Why make a derivative to a naturally occurring substance, you ask?

In the case of DHEA, we have seen its many benefits as a nutritional supplement. Due to the enhanced research on DHEA and the glut of informational material in the form of books, newsletters and the Internet on DHEA, the general public has been buying and taking DHEA in an effort to take advantage of its healing effects.

Some of this supplementation has been under the watchful eye of the patient's health care provider, but unfortunately, a lot is without this guidance. This has led to people taking DHEA in a less than responsible manner, and as I mentioned earlier, sometimes supplementing at very high doses.

Taking DHEA in high doses for a long period of time will result in a higher incidence of adverse reactions. A derivative of DHEA that is more potent and has the same therapeutic benefit but doesn't have the adverse side effects would clearly be an answer to this problem. This derivative would allow patients to essentially take a higher dosage of DHEA for a longer period of time and not have to worry about adverse side effects of virilization, prostate enlargement, etc. It should also be clear by now that in order to receive the maximum health benefits from DHEA, it will have to be taken long-term, and probably at higher doses, to obtain the desired effect for as long as the patient lives.

The other reason that derivatives of naturally occurring substances are important is because of the hormone's action in the body. In order to be truly classified as a "hormone," a substance must have a receptor on a target tissue somewhere in the body. So far, as we have mentioned, DHEA as a parent compound does not have its own receptor. Therefore, if DHEA has an action in our bodies, which it clearly does, it must exert this action via a metabolite or a "derivative" of the parent compound that does have a receptor.

Researchers, such as Dr. Henry Lardy, Vilas Professor Emeritus of Biological Sciences at the University of Wisconsin in Madison, realized this long ago and are actively searching for biologically more active DHEA derivatives that cannot convert to sex steroids. Dr. Lardy is renown for his research on DHEA derivatives and has published over 400 papers in peer-reviewed scientific journals. Dr. Lardy is also a member of the National Academy of Sciences and American Philosophical Society, and has been a member of several scientific advisory councils and served on the editorial boards for many scientific journals.

Dr. Lardy and his team have isolated over 150 DHEA derivatives. In the process of isolating these derivatives, one compound clearly stood out because it provides greater benefits than DHEA. This new derivative is called 7-Keto DHEA.

According to Dr. Lardy, 7-Keto DHEA is more potent than

its parent DHEA and cannot be metabolized to estrogens or testosterone, hence fewer side effects. It is clearly much more beneficial than DHEA and can be taken in high dosages long-term without the risk of serious side effects. Interestingly, 7-Keto DHEA is also a naturally occurring substance and can be found in many of our body tissues. 7-Keto DHEA is now available under the Twin Lab MaxiLIFE™ 7-Keto and 7-Keto Fuel™ brands in health food stores as a revolutionary new dietary supplement.

Scientific Support

Found in all of our bodies, 7-Keto DHEA is a naturally-occurring metabolite of DHEA. I refer you to Figure 13 and please note the oxygen atom in the "7" position of the steroid molecule, which distinguishes it from other metabolites of DHEA.

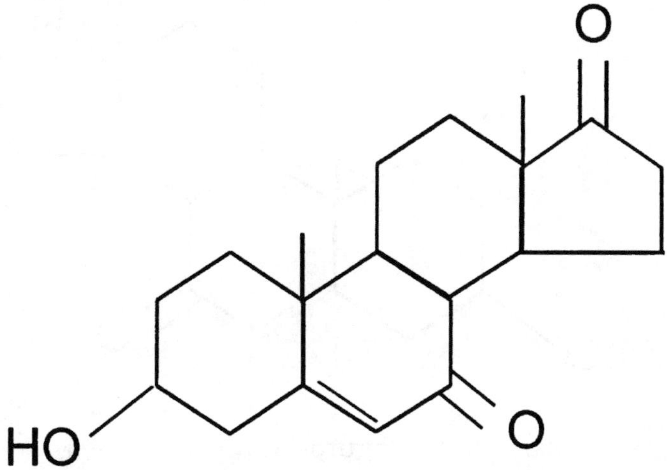

Figure 13.
Chemical Structure of 7-Keto DHEA

The compound 3-Acetyl-7-Keto DHEA can be used as an active form of 7-Keto DHEA. The compound 3-Acetyl-7-Keto DHEA is very similar to 7-Keto DHEA; the only exception is that it contains an acetate group on the "3" position of the steroid molecule which is removed by our bodies upon ingestion. Please see Figure 14, which illustrates the structure of 3-Acetyl-7-Keto DHEA.

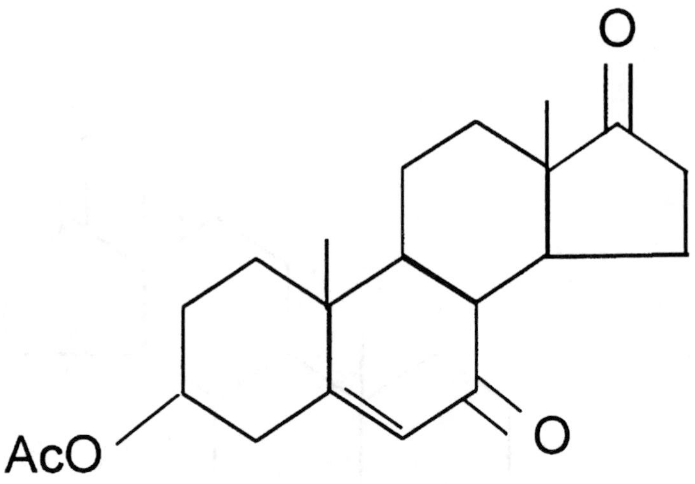

Figure 14.
Chemical Structure of 3-Acetyl-7-Keto DHEA

The acetate group is added to protect the "3" position from oxidation which could occur during synthesis from DHEA in the laboratory. As is the case with other steroid hormones, short chain Acyl esters of 7-Keto DHEA (such as 3-Acetyl-7-Keto DHEA), are readily hydrolyzed by the body by estraces (enzymes) located in the body and tissues, converting it to the naturally occurring compound 7-Keto DHEA.

Therefore, when you buy 7-Keto DHEA from your health food store, what you are getting is the more stable compound 3-Acetyl-7-Keto DHEA, which is later metabolized in your body to 7-Keto DHEA. 7-Keto DHEA then remains the active compound and is not converted to sex hormones, as are other derivatives of DHEA.

Pharmacokinetics of 7-Keto DHEA - Absorption

7-Keto DHEA is absorbed into the bloodstream of humans after oral intake. The absorption characteristics are similar to those of DHEA. Dr. Lardy and others have found that 7-Keto DHEA is rapidly converted to its 3-sulfate derivative just as DHEA is. Maximum levels of this sulfated form occur about two hours after ingestion. This compound is eliminated from the blood at the rate of about 50 percent every two hours.

Pharmacokinetics of 7-Keto DHEA - Distribution

The compound 7-Keto DHEA is found in low concentrations in human blood and tissues, including the brain[32]. Presumably as a result of the 7-Alpha-Hydroxylase enzyme acting on DHEA. Oxidization of DHEA in the body easily produces 7-Keto DHEA. Please see Figure 15 for an outline of steroid metabolism in the body, paying particularly close attention to the conversion of 7-Keto DHEA from its parent compound DHEA.

---

[32] Parker et. al., 1989.

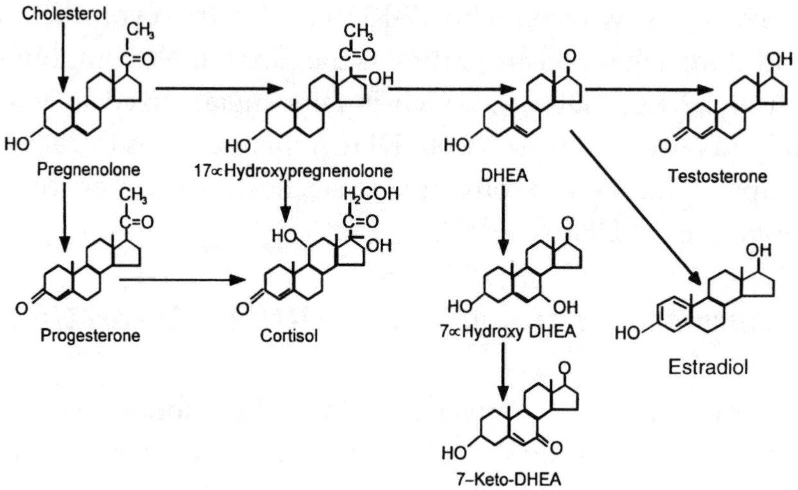

Figure 15.
Outline of Steroid Metabolism of the Adrenal Cortex

Pharmacokinetics of 7-Keto DHEA - Metabolism

Faredin et. al. (1967, 1968) found that enzymes in human skin metabolize DHEA to seven oxygenated derivatives, including 7-Keto DHEA. Numerous rat and other animal studies also prove, without a doubt, that 7-Keto DHEA is a naturally occurring metabolite of DHEA. The exact metabolism of 7-Keto DHEA in the body has not been clearly worked out.

Pharmacokinetics of 7-Keto DHEA - Excretion

7-Keto DHEA is excreted in the urine. This was confirmed by Gallagher (1958). In a Russian study done by Marenich (1979), the urinary excretion of 7-Keto DHEA was studied in 34 healthy men, ranging in age from 20 to 72 years. Maximal excretion was observed between the ages of 20 and 30 years; excretion decreased with advancing age. 7-Keto DHEA is conjugated as a sulfate in the same way prior to excretion as DHEA is.

Mechanism of Action

More than one mode of action for 7-Keto DHEA has been speculated by several different research groups (Lardy, personal conversation, 1997). It has been demonstrated that glucocorticoids antagonize the function of DHEA and of the acetylated form of 7-Keto DHEA. It is postulated that 7-Keto DHEA competes for the receptor that normally functions with glucocorticoids, and vise versa. Therefore, the compound 7-Keto DHEA diminishes the suppression of the immune system by occupying the receptor that normally is activated by glucocorticoids. Since glucocorticoids accomplish an immune system suppression by activating this receptor, 7-Keto DHEA will cause immune system stimulation by antagonizing the glucocorticoid/receptor interaction.

It has been reported that 7-Keto DHEA acts in Simian Immunodeficiency Virus (SIV—akin to HIV/AIDS in humans) by enhancing the production of CD-4 cells. It is known that 7-Keto DHEA enhances the production of the cytokine interleukin-2 (IL-2) in human blood cells. IL-2 stimulates the formation of other cytokines that further activate, along with IL-2, the proliferation of T-cells and promote viral killing.

It is also believed that 7-Keto DHEA has other similar mechanisms of action to that of DHEA, except for those effects mediated through the production of estrogens and testosterone. The compound 7-Keto DHEA has been found in human blood, tissues and urine. The conversion of DHEA to 7-Keto DHEA is the result of a cytochrome P-450 enzyme called 7-Alpha-Hydroxylase and a second enzyme called 7-Dehydrogenase. These two enzymes are found in skin, the adrenal glands, liver, testes and brain tissue.

Safety

7-Keto DHEA has been evalutated in both pre-clinical studies and human clinical trials for safety. The pre-clinical toxicology studies on 7-Keto DHEA were quite favorable. These include a mutagenicity assay to demonstrate no effect on genetic material, an acute rat study and an escalating dose primate study to evaluate short and long-term exposure and tolerance. These studies showed no mutagenic activity and no adverse effects for 7-Keto DHEA up to doses of 2000 mg/kg in rats and 500 mg/kg in primates. It should be noted that 500 mg/kg is approximately 3.5 grams in a normal 70 kg human, which is 70 times greater than the recommended daily dose of approximately 50 mg for humans.

An additional primate study using escalating doses involved groups of three adult monkeys who were fed seven,

35, 70 and 140 mg/kg of 7-Keto DHEA daily. Even at the highest doses for a period of 28 days, no alteration of health or behavior was observed. Blood chemistries remained normal; liver histology was unchanged, as indicated by liver specimens taken before and after the 28-day treatment.

A human clinical trial was also conducted to assess the effects of 7-Keto DHEA on several endocrine and safety parameters in healthy adult men. 7-Keto DHEA was found to be safe and well-tolerated at doses up to 200 mg per day for a 28 day period. The compound lacked any of the clinically significant hormone elevating action that has been reported with DHEA supplementation.

Laboratory safety results also indicated that 7-Keto DHEA does not affect hematology, serum chemistry, or urine values differently than the healthy subjects taking placebo. 7-Keto DHEA did not have detrimental effects and may have had beneficial effects on vital signs and body weight.

The results of these pre-clinical and clinical safety trials indicate that 7-Keto DHEA is a safe and well-tolerated DHEA metabolite which has the potential for use as a supplement in the myriad of medical conditions where DHEA is currently being used.

Efficacy Studies

Dr. Lardy has been the principal researcher investigating the effects of 7-Keto DHEA. Based on his research, Dr. Lardy has been granted several patents on the use of DHEA derivatives, including enhancing or modulating immune function, treatment of Alzheimer's disease and weight loss.

Immunology

Pilot animal studies conducted at the University of Wisconsin at Madison suggest a therapeutic use of 7-Keto DHEA for HIV infected patients with chronic symptoms. Such findings demonstrate effects in increasing CD-4 cell counts in primates chronically infected with Simian Immunodeficiency Virus (SIV) when treated with 7-Keto DHEA. Their levels of total white blood cells increased, as well as their total CD-8 cell counts. Additionally, these SIV infected primates demonstrated improvements in their physical state, their weights increased and their overall behavior and overall clinical condition improved.

Dr. Lardy and his colleagues also demonstrated an increase in antibody production in mice treated with 7- Keto DHEA, compared to DHEA when administered with a Trivalent Influenza Vaccine. This study also demonstrates immune system augmentation by 7-Keto DHEA similar to the Simian studies above.

7-Keto DHEA was also shown to augment Interleukin 2 (IL-2) production in human lymphocytes, in a study done by Nelson et.al. We know that retroviral therapy can suppress HIV replication, but an immune modulator may be necessary to increase the number of CD4 cells (T-helper cells). Numerous injections of IL-2 will increase CD4 cell numbers, but inconvenience and cost limit this treatment modality. In the Nelson study, 7-Keto DHEA was more effective than DHEA at augmenting IL-2 production and deserves further study regarding its uses as an immune modulator in HIV infected patients.

Memory

In a study done by Lardy et.al. at the University of Wisconsin, Madison, 7-Keto DHEA was found to enhance memory in two year old mice. The mice were trained to negotiate a water maze and then were given DHEA or 7-Keto DHEA for comparison purposes. They were re-tested after two weeks. The times to negotiate the maze were significantly shorter with 7-Keto DHEA as opposed to DHEA and the control group. The control mice took 34 seconds; those on DHEA took 22 seconds; and those on 7-Keto DHEA took only 7.6 seconds.

Dr. Lardy found similar results in mice using scopolamine to abolish memory. When protected with 7-Keto DHEA, the mice were able to negotiate the water maze in 6.5 seconds, compared to 11.5 with DHEA treatment and 22 seconds with scopolamine treatment only.

Dr. Lardy performed these studies to assess the use of 7-Keto DHEA in the treatment of memory loss and potentially Alzheimer's disease.

Build Muscle – Lose Fat

7-Keto DHEA could do for physique development what creatine did for sports performance. No exaggeration. I say this for three reasons.

First, you know that muscle growth processes are stimulated as a function of a balance between the body's anabolic hormone levels versus catabolic hormone levels. We often refer to this in an acute state as simply one's testosterone-to cortisol (cortisol is the body's primary stress hormone, reducing total body energy and stimulating catabolism in muscle cells) levels, but we really should make reference to whole body anabolism-promoting and catabolism promoting hormones.

7-Keto DHEA skews the anabolic-to-catabolic ratio in the direction of testosterone-like compounds and away from cortisol. The relatively lower cortisol effects enable the body to build muscle in a growth-promoting environment.

Second, weight control becomes easier with lower relative levels of cortisol, because stress and cortisol itself cause people to eat more. In a study presented at the recent Society of Behavioral Medicine meeting in New Orleans, LA, renowned researchers Kelly Brownell and Elissa Epel found that the more cortisol in a subject's blood stream, the more she ate (specifically high-fat foods).

In their study, 60 women were exposed to deliberately stressful tasks, then allowed to snack without restriction on high-fat or low-fat foods. Subjects' high-fat ingestion rose proportionally with cortisol levels. So, 7-Keto DHEA might also curb your appetite by minimizing cortisol's effects on your body.

Finally, Lardy found that 7-Keto DHEA seems to promote thermogenic activity. Perhaps that's a result of enhanced muscular activity, who knows? The point is, there's another possible fat loss-promoting function of 7-Keto DHEA.

Although information is still being gathered on 7-Keto DHEA, it is apparent that it is light years in front of 95 percent of all other supplements touted to enhance one's health and physique. It has a sound, rational mechanism of action, research to support it, and it's based upon a derivative/isomer paradigm that has worked for decades as the foundation for the development of anabolic steroids (side effects notwithstanding).

The future of health and nutrition lies, in part, in these hormonal alterations and derivatives that produce varying anabolic/androgenic ratios, while minimizing cortisol and enhancing health in a safe and effective manner. This is a very exciting new product because 7-Keto DHEA may be the supplement we've been waiting for to bring all-natural health, fitness and muscular development into the next millennium.

Obesity

In a paper published in the Annals of the New York Academy of Sciences in 1995, Dr. Henry Lardy et. al. described 7-Keto DHEA as a compound that activates thermogenic enzymes in the livers of rats. In fact, the induction potential far exceeded any of the DHEA derivatives tested in that study, indicating increased potency when compared to DHEA. Activation of these thermogenic enzymes is not only an effective assay for activity of DHEA derivatives and can be used as a standard of activity when testing new compounds, it also causes these animals to lose weight without altering their food intake.

Hence, a compound with a high degree of thermogenic enzyme induction such as 7-Keto DHEA would be an excellent weight loss substance. Based on these animal studies, human applications should be pursued.

Skin

In a paper published in 1967 by Faredin et. at., it was proven that DHEA is converted to 7-Keto DHEA by male and female samples of human skin. The exact significance of this finding was not discussed in this article but has since been speculated by others that 7-Keto DHEA may be involved with the normal functioning of hair follicles, sebaceous glands and the normal integrity of the epithelium (skin surface). Further research is needed to prove these findings, but until then, a body of evidence exists supporting a role for 7-Keto DHEA in maintaining the normal healthy state of skin.

Conclusion

This initial data provided by Dr. Lardy and others point to 7-Keto DHEA being a potent immune system stimulator, memory enhancer, anti-obesity agent and a probable skin care additive. What is particularly provocative are the primate studies showing a dramatic improvement in CD-4 cell counts in monkeys infected with SIV, the equivalent of HIV in humans.

If an immune enhancing effect of similar magnitude is found in humans, it would be very complementary to any HIV therapy. It could be a virtual life prolonging therapy for patients infected with AIDS. Human HIV studies are being evaluated, but for now, the preliminary evidence suggests that 7-Keto DHEA could be very beneficial.

7-Keto DHEA in Your Life

As a new dietary supplement, 7-Keto DHEA will augment DHEA in the marketplace. It is a safer and more potent alternative to achieve many of the benefits originally sought from DHEA. 7-Keto DHEA will be manufactured and marketed as a dietary supplement under the provisions of the DSHEA Act. It will be available at most stores that sell dietary supplements throughout the country in a variety of product brands.

In my personal discussions with Dr. Henry Lardy, we discussed the various uses of 7-Keto DHEA. Dr. Lardy believes that this new compound will be able to deliver the same beneficial effects clinically that DHEA does. Certainly, any beneficial effects attributable to DHEA's conversion to estrogens and testosterone will not be present, but all other mechanisms of action will remain intact. He believes the compound to be more potent and better tolerated due to the virtual lack of adverse effects at high dosages.

7-Keto DHEA's potential benefits include up-regulating the body's immune system, providing a protection against disease. In addition, those diseases which have an immunoregulatory cause, such as HIV, systemic lupus erythematosus, multiple sclerosis and rheumatoid arthritis, will very likely show improvement on 7-Keto DHEA, as they did with the parent compound DHEA. I fully anticipate that the other diseases we mentioned in Chapter 3 will also benefit from the long-term use of 7-Keto DHEA such as heart disease, aging, osteoporosis, diabetes mellitus and claudication, to name a few. Ongoing studies at the University of Wisconsin at Madison also reveal memory enhancement in mice after administration of 7-Keto DHEA.

As a cosmetic skin care product, 7-Keto DHEA also promises to be a very beneficial additive. We know from our previous discussions that DHEA is converted to 7-Keto DHEA by skin cells. Skin cells have the required enzyme to catalyze this reaction. This certainly happens for a reason, as do most reactions in our body. It is speculated from previous studies that the natural aging of skin may be linked to declining levels of DHEA as we get older, and that healthy, young appearing skin needs DHEA to maintain its integrity.

Here again, it is not DHEA that exerts this effect, but rather, one of its active metabolites. Since we already know that 7-Keto DHEA is provided to skin cells naturally, why not provide it as a daily topical treatment to keep skin looking young and healthy for a longer period of time. Therefore, we will very likely see many new skin care products introduced to the market with 7-Keto DHEA as a main ingredient. Just think, no more wrinkles!

Personal Experience with 7-Keto DHEA

In order to add as much efficacy and safety information to this new product, I felt it necessary to take it myself. I called the manufacturer and obtained some 7-Keto DHEA that was being used in one of their clinical trials. The capsules were 100 mg each and I began taking one capsule each morning when I got up. The 100 mg dose is higher than suggested of course for daily use but I wanted to see if I experienced any side effects at a high dose, which certainly would make me comfortable prescribing 7-Keto DHEA at 25-50 mg per day.

I was excited, naturally, knowing all the wonderful beneficial effects this compound has since I just completed all the research on it for this book. Four days passed as I took my capsule each morning and I said to myself, "Well, there certainly aren't any terrible side effects." I felt the same as usual but not really any different.

Much to my surprise however, by the fifth and sixth days I started to notice an increase in my energy level. In fact a rather dramatic surge in cognitive alertness and stamina. I loved it! My job is quite demanding during the day with lots of places to be and patients to see and examine.

I found myself looking for more work to do since I was completing my usual duties in less time and really enjoying how quickly my mind was working. At first it didn't occur to me that the 7-Keto DHEA was producing these effects, but as I thought about it, I really did feel a lot different than I usually did. I normally have a good energy level but I actually found myself wanting to run up the stairs instead of taking the elevator. I was ecstatic that this compound could deliver results like these.

What really convinced me though that 7-Keto DHEA was just not another caffeine substitute or multiple vitamin, was the effect it had on a facial infection that I had. Coincidentally before taking 7-Keto DHEA I had been trying to treat a facial eruption on the left side of my jaw. When it first appeared three months previously I told myself it was some type of infection, like acne, since it was red, raised and tender.

Usually when I get these I take a common antibiotic and it disappears in five days or so. So I did what I normally do and took an antibiotic but after 10 days, nothing was happening and in fact it was getting worse. So I said to myself, "You must have picked the wrong antibiotic, try a different, stronger one." So I did and when the second antibiotic failed, I tried a third one and it too offered me no relief. It was then a month since I started treatment and my face looked worse than ever and my wife was urging me to see a dermatologist.

But I rejected the idea because, after all I am a doctor and I should be able to diagnose and heal a simple infection. I was frustrated. I figured if it wasn't bacterial, and not responding to antibiotics, it was probably of fungal origin so I tried an anti-fungal medicine for seven days. Interestingly, there was some improvement but it was not totally healed and in fact was getting rather well established with a hard "knot" below the surface of my skin overlying my jaw. By this time I was getting scared and decided I should see one of my colleagues.

This is about the time I started the 7-Keto DHEA. I was off all other medications and was just taking 100 mg of 7-Keto DHEA every day. I had been on the compound for 10 days when I noticed one morning in the mirror that my jaw wasn't red anymore. I felt it and the "knot" was getting smaller. I smiled into the mirror and said, "It must be the 7-Keto DHEA that is doing this wonderful thing." I was amazed, I knew that 7-Keto DHEA could up-regulate my immune system but this was a pretty convincing example that I couldn't quite believe. I decided to stop the 7-Keto DHEA to see what would happen.

I was literally shocked and quite frankly astonished to see my face getting worse each day I was off the compound. By the fifth day, my jaw was red, tender and the "knot" had returned with a vengeance. I looked in the mirror on the morning of the seventh day and said, "There's only one way to bring this reaction to a screeching halt." I started taking the 7-Keto DHEA again and by the fourth day my face was healing.

I have now been taking 7-Keto DHEA for two and one-half months, my face has totally healed and I feel physically rejuvenated. I am so pleased with the experience of taking 7-Keto DHEA, I can honestly testify that I experience no adverse side effects. I am also now wondering if the compound isn't more potent than I originally thought and am convinced that it stimulates the immune system to fight infections.

In conclusion, with 7-Keto DHEA in your life, you should benefit by being a healthier individual with less chance of serious illness. If you are already afflicted with a chronic disease, 7-Keto DHEA will provide an improvement to your quality of life. Used long-term, it may ameliorate the effects of aging, particularly to your skin, and possibly enhance memory. Since it is a safer second generation DHEA derivative, worry free long-term use will be possible via many different delivery modalities.

CHAPTER FIVE

Scientific Parallels - The Vitamin D Story

We are in the midst of a very exciting new trend in natural product research. A trend which may revolutionize the dietary supplement industry. If successful, this research could yield many new and important dietary supplement products to be used as dietary supplements or even pharmaceuticals, if new in-roads to the human endocrine system are discovered. DHEA is actually a low potency natural hormone that has no receptor of its own in the body and has enough negative side effects that it is inappropriate for long-term use. This has led researchers to seek out new derivatives of DHEA, in essence, a search for the "ultimate" hormone.

This is not a new phenomenon in drug research, and in fact, has been used by the pharmaceutical industry for many years. Many of our existing pharmaceuticals, some of which I prescribe to my patients every day, were discovered by derivative research. These agents typically are more potent, have a specific receptor protein in the body, and are more efficacious than their predecessors. What is new about this phenomenon is that it has never been extended to the dietary supplement industry as it is now being applied.

To bring the importance of this kind of research to the forefront and also to provide a similar correlation to DHEA derivative research, I would like to take a moment to tell you the Vitamin D story. Vitamin D and DHEA are both naturally occurring substances in our bodies and both are low potency compounds without specific receptors. They both provide the body with beneficial effects. For Vitamin D, it is the enhancement of calcium and phosphorus absorption, which prevents the disease Rickets, and for DHEA, it is the enhancement of immune system function. Similarly is the fact that Vitamin D is not the active hormone but actually a "pro-hormone," as is DHEA.

The Vitamin D story is an inspiration for all researchers looking for the truth and striving to find the answers to the very tough questions of the universe. The story was told to me by Dr. Hector DeLuca, as I sat in his office at the University of Wisconsin at Madison. Dr. DeLuca is the Chairman of the Biochemistry Department at the University of Wisconsin at Madison and the discoverer of the active form of Vitamin D.

Dr. DeLuca feels it is indeed rare and unexpected when an investigation of basic science, like that needed to find the active form of Vitamin D, has such an immediate and practical application to clinical medicine. He also feels that the similarities between what happened with Vitamin D and what is now happening with DHEA are strikingly historic, and that further research by Dr. Lardy may indeed yield the "ultimate" hormone. Dr. DeLuca is now past middle-age and his many years of experience in biochemistry research are reflected in his confident voice. He has a kind face and mannerisms I've come to expect from the many professors I have known in my career. He sat back in his chair, smiled and I sat expectantly on the other side of his desk. The Vitamin D story started as the sun of a beautiful June afternoon shown through his office windows. The Vitamin D story flowed as if he had told it a million times, I took notes and this is what I learned.

The Search for Solutions

From 1919 through 1924, the discovery of Vitamin D and its production in skin and foods by ultraviolet irradiation led to the elimination of Rickets as a major medical problem. Rickets is the Vitamin D deficiency disease of the young. In the late 1800's and the beginning of this century, this disease appeared in epidemic proportions in Northern Europe, North America and Northern Asia.

Sir Edward Mellanby demonstrated Rickets to be at least in part a nutritional disorder that he could heal with cod liver oil. McCollum demonstrated that the healing factor in cod liver oil was a new vitamin called Vitamin D. Huldshinsky and his coworkers also demonstrated that Rickets could be healed by ultraviolet light. Steenbock, putting together both the nutritional and ultraviolet light concepts, demonstrated that ultraviolet light induced the Vitamin D compound in the fatty portions of diet and of skin. By irradiating food, Steenbock provided the means whereby Rickets could be eliminated as a major medical problem.

This basic work also provided the means whereby chemists could isolate and identify the structure of Vitamin D, which led ultimately to the chemical synthesis of large amounts of the compound. Vitamin D therefore became available to the physician for pharmacological treatment of many metabolic bone diseases. Thus, before the 1940's basic investigations of Vitamin D provided the medical world with important new advances in the treatment of metabolic bone disease.

Rickets and osteomalacia, the Vitamin D deficiency diseases, are characterized by a failure of the organic matrix to acquire the hydroxyapatite mineral. The absence of this mineral leaves the collagen fibrils in a soft and pliable state that gives rise to the overt symptoms of Rickets, which are basically soft bones. The presence of adequate amounts of calcium and phosphorus in plasma therefore brings about the normal bone growth and mineralization, and Vitamin D plays a role in this process. Vitamin D brings about the elevation of plasma calcium and phosphorus by these three basic mechanisms:

1. It is the only substance known that stimulates the enterocytes of the small intestine to transport calcium from the lumen to the plasma compartment. In the same cells, it brings about the transport of phosphorus into the plasma compartment as well.

2. Because the presence of calcium in the diet, and hence the intestine, is not predictable, the body utilizes the skeleton as a ready source of calcium. To mobilize calcium from the skeleton, two hormones working in concert are involved: Vitamin D and parathyroid hormone.

3. In the distal renal tubules of the kidney, calcium is reabsorbed from the urine back into the plasma under the influence of parathyroid hormone and Vitamin D, and therefore calcium levels increase in the plasma.

Plasma calcium and phosphorus are elevated because of these three mechanisms, and thus new bone is mineralized.

The next important development in the Vitamin D story was the discovery that it must be metabolized before becoming an active form. During the 1950's and early 1960's until 1967, it was thought that Vitamin D must be active directly without further modification. We now know, however, that Vitamin D must first be 25-Hydroxylated in the liver, and subsequently 1-μ-Hydroxylated in the kidney before it can carry out the classical functions described above.

This idea was first described in 1966 by Dr. DeLuca when he noted that the Vitamin D molecule must be modified before it could function to elevate blood calcium, a discovery resulting from early metabolic work. Vitamin D-3 is the compound produced in the skin by the absorption of ultraviolet light by 7-Dehydrocholesterol, found normally in the skin. This photochemical process is so extremely efficient that only as much as ten minutes of summer sun on the hands and face is sufficient to produce ten micrograms of Vitamin D-3 or 400 IU, the recommended daily allowance for most human beings.

Further work led to the discovery of the liver-produced 25-Hydroxy Vitamin D which, for a time, was believed to be the functional form of Vitamin D-3. In 1971, the active form of Vitamin D was isolated from a target organ, the intestine, and was chemically identified as1-μ-25-Dihydroxyvitamin D-3.

It was at this time that Dr. DeLuca made this discovery by theorizing that the active form of Vitamin D-3 must be present at the intestinal level, since this is where calcium absorption takes place. Therefore, he would be able to find the active compound at its receptor site in the intestine.

He was correct! He was able to isolate two micrograms of a polar metabolite, which later became known as 1-μ-25-Dihydroxyvitamin D-3, the active form of Vitamin D-3. It was later discovered that the active form of Vitamin

D-3 originated in the kidney but had its action in the intestine and bone. Eventually, the amino acid sequence (protein structure) of the 1-μ-25 Dihydroxyvitamin D-3 receptor was discovered in the intestine, and for the first time, Vitamin D-3 became a hormone and an integral part of the human endocrine system. Most important was the later discovery that the production of 1-μ-25 Dihydroxyvitamin D-3 is feedback regulated by serum calcium through the parathyroid glands, clearly defining the Vitamin D-based endocrine system.

Our discussions about Vitamin D drifted to some of its uses that are just now starting to be explored in addition to the treatment of Vitamin D resistant Rickets, renal osteodystrophy and osteoporosis. Some of these examples include Vitamin D as a regulator of insulin secretion or as a hormone causing the differentiation of promyelocytes to monocytes or macrophages. The Vitamin D receptor has been found to exist in 60 percent or more of all cancer cell lines and we talked about the theoretical possibilities of active Vitamin D suppressing these tumors in pharmacological amounts.

Lastly, several groups of researchers have speculated that 1-Alpha-25 Dihydroxyvitamin D-3 may be useful in the treatment of psoriasis due to its suppressive effects on the keratinocytes of human skin. The possible uses seem endless and Dr. DeLuca feels there are more to come, especially in the area of autoimmune diseases.

To further illustrate his point, Dr. DeLuca briefly described the past and current research focused on Vitamin A and its derivatives. Here again is a compound without a receptor in the body, where through basic science research has been studied and found to have active derivatives.

Retinoic acid is a particularly active form of Vitamin A with its own receptor, and now has very wide-spread use with ongoing research to future positive effects as an anticancer drug.

The New Frontier

After listening to Dr. DeLuca, I was very excited to think that what happened to Vitamin D could very easily happen to DHEA. The correlation between the two compounds is amazingly similar in almost every respect.

I could not help but think that Dr. Lardy's compound, 7-Keto DHEA, is the equivalent of 25-hydroxyvitamin D-3, a stepping stone to the discovery of the active form of DHEA, just as of 25-hydroxyvitamin D-3 was the precursor to finding 1-μ-25 Dihydroxyvitamin D-3, the active form of Vitamin D. Once the active form of DHEA is discovered and its receptor is localized and identified, new uses and potential benefits of the new compound will come to light, just as they did with Vitamin D.

What is even more important, however, is that this type of research into derivatives of naturally occurring substances, is currently in its infancy. The potential benefits, should researchers like Dr. Lardy, Dr. DeLuca and others be allowed to continue their work, are astronomical. New, exciting compounds with benefits heretofore undiscovered will be introduced, and answers to questions previously unknown will seem obvious. This new frontier within the dietary supplement industry is vital to these future discoveries, and hopefully will continue and flourish.

CHAPTER SIX

BoomerAge:
Enhancing The Model

We are witnessing the integration of complementary medical care into our existing conventional medical system. The BoomerAge Model of health delivery is finally upon us. As a BoomerDoc I feel it is now necessary to embrace this concept of integration. As one of many BoomerDocs I have come to understand the wisdom behind integrating conventional care with complementary care.

I also feel that as BoomerDocs we need to take it upon ourselves to listen to our patients and enhance the model. Over time the model will evolve with our help and the help of the complementary practitioners and we will see improved outcomes, an emphasis on safety, and patients who are happy and more involved with their care than ever before.

The time has finally come for people to benefit from both systems of health care delivery. No longer do patients have to rely only on their medical doctors for treatment of their diseases. No longer will I, as a practicing physician, be limited to treatments within the allopathic medical system. My patients will be happier and healthier, and have a better quality of life than they ever did before.

The opportunities for self-help will explode. With the proper information and guidance, the use of these therapies should eventually decrease the amount of money spent for health care. There is no reason why these two systems of health care delivery cannot be integrated, especially when the focus is on the appropriate care of sick people.

The real focus of modern medicine has been lost. No longer are the patients more important than the "bottom line." Medicine is now "big business." The public is well aware of this, which is one of the reasons they are going out on their own, and in larger and larger numbers, seeking out health care alternatives other than conventional medicine. They are desperately seeking someone who will whole-heartedly listen to their problems, comfort them and then provide them with as many options for treatment as possible. These treatments, I have discovered, are not only to cure or treat their disease, but also to provide comfort, a better quality of life and peace of mind.

Complementary medical care provides many of these important treatments, and those of us in the conventional medical field should stand up, take notice and embrace these principles of care. We are treating only a small part of our patients' problems and we are not listening to what they really want. This integration is urgently needed and represents a new model for health care in our country.

The evolution of DHEA and its derivatives has led to the introduction of 7-Keto DHEA as a dietary supplement and skin care product. As we have mentioned, the search for derivatives of naturally occurring substances is fueled by the curiosity of why and how the parent compound exerts its action on the body. Many parent compounds do not have their own receptor in the body and are low potency requiring high doses to exert their effects. Rather, it is an active metabolic derivative, which is the real hormone and the responsible compound for the body's beneficial effect.

In the search for more active derivatives of DHEA, a

highly potent and safe second generation DHEA derivative was discovered. This compound, called 7-Keto DHEA, is the first of its kind to be introduced to the marketplace.

As a derivative of a naturally occurring substance, 7-Keto DHEA is paving the way for future research on many other natural substances. I cannot stress enough what an important development this is. Not only have Dr. Lardy and his colleagues developed an active more potent derivative of DHEA with less side effects, they have opened our eyes and our minds to the possibility of future derivatives of naturally occurring substances.

Just think of all the possible beneficial compounds that could be developed if this research is continued and directed properly. Many of the complementary therapies we take every day could be made better, more effective, and possibly have less side effects than their parent compounds.

Maybe, and this has been a dream of my own, one of these new derivative compounds will serendipitously provide a cure for the common cold, lupus or some types of cancers. Hopefully, researchers like Dr. Lardy will be given the support they need to aggressively seek out these new compounds, and we as consumers will be given the chance to benefit from their discoveries.

As derivative research continues in the future, the process of development and discovery of 7-Keto DHEA will provide a standard by which other derivatives will be sought. Certainly 7-Keto DHEA's purity and safety profile will also set a new standard of excellence against which all other derivatives will be judged. This is truly a landmark discovery and as consumers, we are certainly lucky to be able to benefit by having a more potent DHEA derivative supplement that does not increase sex hormones.

Research like that needed to design 7-Keto DHEA is one example of how complementary medicine is contributing to the well being of many individuals. Consumers should encourage researchers to continue to develop safe products to complement allopathic medicine and provide greater options for self-care. This new derivative research is certainly provocative and hopefully will provide us with many new compounds in the future.

In conclusion, the BoomerAge Model of integrated health care is a concept born at a time when consumers are looking for more options for their health and well-being. The Boomers have been a driving force behind the model, hence the name. They, as a group, are challenging the conventional medical system to think creatively and make this integration happen.

BoomerDocs need to be as receptive as possible, listen to their patients, educate themselves about complementary care, support the use of complementary methods of healing and help to provide the scientific substantiation that the new system will need as it evolves. It is an exciting new concept and there is much to learn and much to do.

Glossary

ACTH: Adrenocorticotropic hormone which is a pituitary hormone that acts on the adrenal gland for the purpose of stimulating the production of steroids, such as epinephrine, cortisol and DHEA.

ADH: Antidiuretic hormone. A substance produced by the posterior section of the pituitary gland which suppresses the rate of urine formation in the body.

Acetyl: A monovalent radical with a chemical structure CH3CO.

Acetylation: The introduction of an acetyl group in the molecule of an organic compound.

Acyl Ester: An organic radical derived from an organic acid by removal of the hydroxyl (OH) group.

Acupuncture: The Chinese practice of piercing specific peripheral nerves with needles to relieve the discomfort associated with painful disorders, to induce surgical anesthesia or for other therapeutic purposes.

Adrenal Gland: An endocrine gland that lies atop each kidney, responsible for the production of DHEA and other steroids.

Addison's Disease: A disease characterized by a bronze-like pigmentation of the skin, progressive anemia, low blood pressure, diarrhea and digestive disturbances due to hypo-functioning of the adrenal glands, which is usually fatal if unrecognized.

Agonist: A chemical which stimulates a specific receptor in a positive manner, resulting in a bodily reaction normally triggered by that receptor.

Allopathic Medicine: A term usually used to describe our present system of therapeutics in which diseases are treated by producing a condition incompatible with, or antagonistic to the condition to be cured or alleviated.

Alzheimer's Disease: A type of irreversible dementia where there is a progressive degeneration of nerve cells in the brain, resulting in memory loss, disorientation, mood changes and confusion.

Amylase: An enzyme that catalyzes the hydrolysis of starch into smaller molecules. Amylase is usually produced by the pancreas and/or the salivary glands.

Androstenediol: An intermediate steroid produced from DHEA which functions as an androgen in the body and is eventually metabolized to testosterone and estrogens derivatives.

Androstenetriol: An intermediate steroid produced from DHEA which functions as an androgen in the body and is eventually metabolized to testosterone and estrogens derivatives.

Anemia: A reduction below normal in the number of red blood cells in the body occurring either from blood loss, iron deficiency or other causes.

Antagonist: A chemical which interacts with a receptor in a negative manner resulting in a bodily reaction opposite that usually produced by that particular receptor.

Antibody: A soluble protein molecule produced and secreted by B-cells in response to an antigen (foreign substance), which is capable of binding to that specific antigen.

Antigen: Any substance that stimulates an immune system response with an antibody. Examples would be bacteria, viruses and other foreign proteins.

Antioxidant: A substance that protects the body against damaging free radicals. Examples of antioxidants would be Vitamin C, Vitamin E, Beta carotene and coenzyme Q-10.

Arteriosclerotic Heart Disease: A disease characterized by the thickening and loss of elasticity of the arterial walls of the coronary arteries of the heart. This often results in a decreased flow of blood through the coronary arteries, which may result in a heart attack.

Basophil: A type of white blood cell involved in the process of fighting infections in the body.

Bell's Palsy: Facial paralysis due to a lesion or constriction of the facial nerve, usually resulting in a characteristic distortion of the face.

Bioelectromagnetic: The study of the role of electromagnetic impulses on biological organisms.

Biofeedback: The process of providing visual or auditory evidence to a person of the status of an autonomic body function, as by the sounding of a tone when blood pressure is at a desirable level so that he or she may exert control over that function. This training takes place at a subconscious level as well as a conscious level of awareness.

Biosynthesis: A process of building up a chemical compound using the physiologic processes of a living organism.

Capitated Medical Systems: A type of medical insurance where providers of medical services are paid a single fee for each person within the system without regard to their medical condition.

Chiropractic: A system of therapeutics based upon the claim that diseases caused by abnormal function of the nervous system. It attempts to restore normal function of the nervous system by manipulation and treatment of the structures of the human body, especially those of the spinal column.

Cholesterol: A fatty steroid substance in the body made by the liver or absorbed from the diet. Cholesterol is commonly found in animal fats and oils; also milk, egg yolks and organ meats. It is a very important steroid in the body needed to make bile and other steroid hormones, particularly DHEA.

Circadian Rhythm: A term usually used to describe the rhythmic repetition of certain phenomenon in living organisms occurring during a 24 hour period. An example of a circadian rhythm would be the usual production of high amounts of cortisol during the early morning hours each day in human beings.

Claudication: A complex of symptoms characterized by the absence of pain or discomfort in a limb when at rest, the commencement of pain, tension and weakness after walking is begun, intensification of the condition until walking becomes impossible, and the disappearance of symptoms after a period of rest. The condition is usually seen in occlusive arterial diseases of the lower extremities.

Complementary Medicine: A term used today to describe a system of therapeutics encompassing most all therapies except allopathic medicine. this would include treating patients with acupuncture, chiropractic, massage therapy, etc.

Cytochrome P450: An enzyme found in the liver whose primary function is electron transport causing the metabolism of hormones and some medications in the body.

Cytokine: A hormone secreted by various immune cells, including T-cells and macrophages. Cytokines act as messengers within the immune system of the body. Examples include interleukin and interferon.

Cytosol: The liquid medium of the cytoplasm of the cell. The cytoplasm of a cell is basically the entire contents of a specific cell exclusive of the nucleus. The cytosol would, therefore, be the cytoplasm minus the organelles and nonmembranous insoluble components of the cytoplasm.

Demyelination: To destroy or remove the myelin sheath of a nerve or nerves.

Diabetes Mellitus: A metabolic disorder in which the ability to oxidize carbohydrates is more or less completely lost, usually due to faulty pancreatic activity, resulting in a lack of insulin. This produces high levels of blood sugar, resulting in symptoms of thirst, hunger and weakness.

Duodenum: The upper portion of the small intestine that connects the lower part of the stomach to the jejunum. The duodenum is important since many of our digestive processes occur in the duodenum, along with the absorption of nutrients.

Endocrine: A system of hormone secretion applied to organs whose function is to directly secrete their hormones into the blood stream to interact with a specific target organ or tissue.

Endogenous: Growing from within. Developing or originating within the organism or arising from causes within the organism.

Enterocytes: A term used to describe the cells lining the small intestine whose primary function is nutrient absorption.

Enzymes: A protein capable of accelerating or producing by catalytic action some change in a substrate for which is often specific. Enzymes in the body are divided into several different groups, depending on their actions, and they are quite useful in the synthesis and breakdown of many of our body's hormones and other chemicals.

Eosinophils: A type of white blood cell typically involved in the process of fighting parasitic infections in the body, or reacting to allergic phenomenon affecting the body.

Epstein Barr Virus: A herpes virus originally isolated from Burkitt lymphomas and believed to be the causative agent of infectious mononucleosis.

Etiology: The study or theory of the factors that cause disease and the method of their introduction to the host.

Exocrine: A process of hormone secretion whereby a gland secretes its hormone via a specific duct which in turn connects to the target tissue. It is the opposite of an endocrine gland secretion, since it does not secrete its hormones directly into the bloodstream.

FSH: Follicle stimulating hormone. One of the gonadotropic hormones of the anterior pituitary, which stimulates the growth and maturation of specific follicles within the ovary. It also stimulates the production of sperm in the male.

Feedback loop: A process used for regulation of hormone function in the body. It basically is the return of some of the output of a system as input, so as to exert some control of the process of affecting the ultimate outcome.

GH: Growth hormone. A substance that stimulates growth in the body and is secreted by the anterior pituitary gland.

Geriatric: That branch of medicine which treats all problems peculiar to old age and the aging process.

Glucocorticoid: Any corticoid substance which increases glyconeogenesis, which is the process of raising the concentration of liver glycogen and blood sugar. In man the most important glucocorticoids are cortisol and corticosterone. Glucocorticoids also influence fat and protein metabolism, help maintain arterial blood pressure and also inhibit inflammatory and allergic responses.

HDL: High density lipoprotein (good cholesterol).

Herbs/Herbalism: A therapeutic process using leafy plants without woody stems in the treatment of disease.

Hirsutism: A process describing abnormal hair growth, especially in women.

Homeopathy: A system of therapeutics founded by Samuel Hahnemann (1755-1843) in which diseases are treated by drugs which are capable of producing in healthy persons symptoms like those of the disease to be treated, the drug being administered in very minute doses.

Hormone: A chemical substance produced in the body by an organ, or cells of an organ, which has a specific regulatory affect on the activity of a certain target tissue.

Hypnosis: An artificially induced passive state in which there is increased amenability and responsiveness to suggestions and commands, provided that these do not conflict seriously with the subjects' own conscious or unconscious wishes.

Hypothalamus: A gland located in the brain which has a stimulatory affect on the pituitary gland, also located in the brain. The hypothalamus, therefore, plays a role in water balance, body temperature, sleep, food intake and the development of secondary sex characteristics.

Hypothyroidism: A deficiency of thyroid activity. In adults it is most common in women and is characterized by a decrease in basometabolic rate, tiredness and a sensitivity to cold.

Immune System: A system in the body used to fight particular diseases using antibodies created to challenge certain antigens in addition to direct killing of foreign substances using specific "killer" cells, which are part of the immune system.

Inderal: A trade name describing a generic product called Propranolol. Propranolol is a beta blocker medication used for many different disease processes, including the treatment of hypertension, arteriosclerotic heart disease and migraine headaches.

Infectious Mononucleosis: An acute infectious disease associated with the Epstein Barr Virus and characterized by fever, malaise, sore throat, enlargement of lymph nodes and spleen with atypcial lymphocytes (white blood cells) noted on peripheral blood smears in the laboratory.

Interferon: A type of cytokine that kills viruses by inhibiting the creation of viral RNA and proteins. There are three types of interferons: alpha, beta and gamma.

Interleukin: A group of cytokines produced by the immune system, particularly the T-cells, in response to antigenic stimulation. These are soluble substances responsible for stimulating, suppressing and orchestrating the activities of the immune system, thus maintaining the communication pathways among cells and tissues. An example of an interleukin is interleukin-2, which is produced by CD-4 cells, which alerts the immune systems that a foreign substance has breached the defenses and signals other interleukins and interferons to activate the production of T-cells and B-cells necessary to mount an attack against that invader.

Keratinocytes: The epidermal cell which synthesizes keratin, which is the principal constituent of skin, hair and nails.

Kidney: One of two organs in the body whose main purpose is to filter the blood, excreting the end products of body metabolism in the form of urine.

LDL: Low density lipoprotein (bad cholesterol).

LH: Luteinizing hormone, a gonadotropic hormone of the anterior pituitary gland which acts with the follicle stimulating hormone to cause ovulation of mature follicles in the ovary and secretion of estrogens by the ovary as well.

Lanoxin: A trade name of a generic product called Digoxin. Digoxin is a cardiotonic glycoside obtained from the leaves of the plant Digitalis lanata, which is used in the treatment of congestive heart failure.

Leukocyte: A generic term used to describe white blood cells in the body.

Libido: The desire for sexual activity.

Lymphocyte: A type of white blood cell, which is a small cell found in the blood lymph and lymphoid tissue. Lymphocytes are an important part of the body's immune system. Both B-and T-cells are types of lymphocytes which become activated when they come in contact with antigens in the body.

Macrobiotics: A term used to describe a type of diet consisting of 60 percent whole grain cereals, 25 percent vegetables, ten percent beans and sea vegetables and five percent soups. No macrobiotic diet includes meat or poultry.

Macrophage: A large and versatile immune cell that when stimulated destroys foreign substances by engulfing them through a process called phagocytosis. Their function also is as an important source of immune secretions.

Melatonin: A hormone synthesized by the pineal gland.

Metabolic Conjugate: A process of metabolism which causes a coupling of two substances.

Metabolite: Any substance produced by metabolism or by a metabolic process. Metabolism is basically the sum of all the physical and chemical processes by which any living organized substance is produced and maintained (anabolism), and also the transformation by which energy is made available for the uses of the organism (catabolism).

Mineralocorticoid: A corticoid particularly effective in causing the retention of sodium and the loss of potassium.

Molecule: The smallest amount of a specific chemical substance that can exist alone. (To break a molecule down into its constant atoms is to change its character; a molecule of water, for example, reverts to oxygen and hydrogen.)

Monocyte: Another type of immune cell that is formed in the bone marrow and lives in the blood for about 24 hours. After that time, a monocyte travels to various organs and eventually evolves into a macrophage.

Myocardial Infarction: A process resulting in the death of myocardial (heart) tissue. This is usually the result of the interruption of the blood supply to that particular area, as in occlusion of a coronary artery.

Opportunistic Infection: An infection in an immunosuppressed person caused by an organism that does not usually trouble people with healthy immune systems.

Osteoblast: A cell which arises from a fibroblast and which, as it matures, is associated with the production of bone.

Osteoclast: A large multi-nuclear cell associated with the absorption and removal of bone.

Oxidation: The active oxidizing, or state of being oxidized. Chemically, it consists in the increase of positive charges on an atom or the loss of negative charges. Most biological oxidations are accomplished by the removal of a pair of hydrogen atoms (dehydrogenation) from a molecule.

Oxytocin: One of two hormones formed by the cells of the hypothalamus and stored in the posterior lobe of the pituitary gland. The other hormone is ADH, described early. Oxytocin stimulates the contraction of the uterine musculature. When it is prepared synthetically it can be used to induce active labor in humans.

PMN: Polymorphonuclear neutrophil, which basically is another term for leukocyte, or white blood cell.

PTH: Parathyroid hormone. A hormone produced by the parathyroid gland involved in the metabolism of calcium and phosphorus in the body.

Pancreas: A large, elongated organ located in the mid-abdomen which is both an endocrine and exocrine gland for the body. It secretes a variety of digestive enzymes, in addition to insulin.

Pharmacokinetics: The study of the action of a drug in the body over a period of time, including the processes of absorption, distribution, localization in tissues, biotrasnformation and excretion.

Pineal Gland: A small gland in the brain responsible for secreting melatonin and serotonin, both of which help to control the body's time clock, appetite and mood.

Pituitary Gland: A gland located at the base of the brain, which is called the master gland and is essentially responsible for the control of all the other glands in the body. Pituitary gland is responsible for the secretion of important stimulatory hormones, such as ACTH, which stimulates the adrenal gland to produce DHEA.

Placebo: An inactive substance or preparation given to satisfy the patients' symbolic need for drug therapy and used in controlled studies to determine the efficacy of medicinal substances. A placebo typically has no intrinsic therapeutic value.

Platelet: A very small cell in the bloodstream, found in all mammals, chiefly known for its role in blood coagulation. It is also called a thrombocyte.

Pregnenolone: A corticosteroid which is a direct metabolic derivative of cholesterol and can be subsequently metabolized to progesterone and DHEA. It has been used as a anti-arthritic; also has been used to relieve fatigue caused by stress.

Promyelocyte: A precursor of leukocytes formed in the bone marrow. It is an intermediate cell in the development between a myeloblast and a myelocyte.

Prostate Gland: A gland in the male which surrounds the neck of the bladder and the urethra. It consists of a median lobe and two lateral lobes, and has ducts which empty into the urethra. The prostate basically contributes the liquid portion of seminal fluid.

Receptor: A specific chemical grouping on the surface of an immunologically competent cell with the capability of combining specifically with an antigen or a stimulatory substance.

Renal Osteodystrophy: A condition resulting from a chronic disease of the kidneys with its onset usually in childhood. It is characterized by impaired renal function, elevated serum phosphorus and low serum calcium levels. The resultant bone disease is basically osteomalacia, which is a condition marked by the softening of bones due to impaired mineralization.

Serotonin: A vasoconstrictor chemical found in serum and many body tissues produced by the pineal gland.

Steroid: A chemical compound with a characteristic multiple ring structure. All human steroids are made from the parent compound cholesterol and are manufactured in various organs throughout the body. Some of the substances included in this group are progesterone, DHEA, estrogens and cortisol derivatives.

Substrate: A substance upon which an enzyme acts.

Synthesis: The artificial building up of a chemical compound by the union of its elements or from other suitable starting materials.

T-Cells: Small white blood cells that orchestrate and/or directly participate in the immune defenses. Also known as T-lymphocytes, they are processed in the thymus and secrete lymphokines.

TNF: Tumor necrosis factor.

TRH: Thyrotropic hormone, also called thyrotropin. A hormone produced by the hypothalamus to stimulate the pituitary gland to produce TSH.

TSH: Thyroid stimulating hormone. A hormone produced by the pituitary gland to stimulate the thyroid gland to produce thyroid hormone.

Thymus Gland: A ductless, gland-like body situated in the anterior mediastinal cavity which reaches maximum development during the early years of childhood and then undergoes involution. Once considered an endocrine gland, it is now thought to be a lymphoid body. It is now a site of lymphocyte production and plays a role in immunologic competence.

Triglycerides: A compound consisting of three molecules of fatty acid esterified to glycerol. It is a neutral fat synthesized from carbohydrates for storage inhuman fat cells.

Units of Measure: For the purposes of discussion, we will briefly discuss metric weights.

> 1 kilogram = 1,000 grams
>
> 1 gram = 1,000 milligrams
>
> 1 milligram = 1,000 micrograms
>
> 1 liter = 1,000 cc's
>
> 30 cc's = 1 ounce
>
> 1 deciliter (dl) = 100 cc's (1 ml = 1 cc)

VLDL: Very low density lipoprotein.

Vitamins: A general term for a number of unrelated organic substances that occur in many foods in small amounts and that are necessary for the normal metabolic functioning of the body. They may be water soluble or fat soluble.

Bibliography

Chapter 2

Eisenberg, D.M.; Kessler, R.C. et. al., Unconventional Medicine in the United States, New England Journal of Medicine, 1993, 378:246-252.

Dietary Supplement Health and Education Act of 1994 (1994) Pub. L. No. 103-417, 108 Stat. 4325 (1994).

Chapter 3

Adlercreutz, H.; Kerstell, J.; Schaumann, K.O. et. al. Plasma lipids and steroid hormones in patients with hypercholesterolemia or hyperlipidemia during dehydroepiandrosterone sulphate administration. Europ. J. Clin. Invest. 1972; 2:91-95.

Apfelbaum, M.; Bishop, J.S.; Cressey, D. et. al., Human or murine endocrine and metabolic rhythms after changes in meal timing with or without a fixed activity schedule. Prog. 56th Meeting Endo. Soc. A-209, 1974; abst. 308.

Barrett-Connor, E.; Khaw, K.T.; Yen, S.S.C. A prospective study of dehydroepiandrosterone sulfate, mortality and cardiovascular disease. New England Journal of Medicine, 1986; 315:1519-24.

Barrett-Connor, E.; Khaw, K.T. Absence of an inverse relation of dehydroepiandrosterone sulfate with cardiovascular mortality in postmenopausal women. N.E.J.M. 1987; 317:711.

Bates, G.W., Jr.; Egerman, R.S.; Umstot, E.S. et. al. DHEA attenuates study induced declines in insulin sensitivity in postmenopausal women. Ann. NY Acad. Sci. 1995; 774:291-3.

Chatterton, R.T.; Green, D.; Harris, S. et. al. Longitudinal study of adrenal steroids in a cohort of HIV infected patients with hemophilia. J. Lab. Clin. Med. 1996; 127:545-52.

Christeff, N.; Michon, C.; Goertz, G. et. al. Abnormal free fatty acids and cortisol concentrations in the serum of AIDS patients. Eur. J. Cancer Clin. Oncol. 1988; 24:1179-83.

Cleary, M.P.; Shepherd, A.; Zisk, J. et. al. Effect of dehydroepiandrosterone on body weight and food intake in rats. Nutr. Behav. 1983; 1:127-136.

Clerici, M.; Shearer, G.M. A TH-1 to TH-2 switch is a critical step in the etiology of HIV infection. Immunol. Today 1993; 14:107-111.

Clerici, M.; Bevilacqua, M.; Vago, T. et. al. An immunoendro-crinological hypothesis of HIV infection. Lancet 1994; 343:1552-53.

DePrato, R.A.; Rothschild, J. The AIDS virus as an opportunistic organism inducing a state of chronic relative cortisol excess: therapeutic implications. Med. Hypotheses 1986; 21:253-66.

DePeretti, E.; Forest, M.G. Pattern of plasma dehydroepiandrosterone sulfate levels in humans from birth to adulthood: evidence for testicular production: Jnl. Clin. Endocrino. Metab., 1978; 47:571-77.

Farendin, I.; Toth, I.; Fazekas, A.G. et. al. The in-vitro metabolism of [4-14C] androst-4-ene-3, 17-dione by normal and hirsute female skin. Int. J. Dermatol., 1970; 9:147-52.

Fullerton, D.T.; Wenzel, F.J.; Lohrena, F.N. et al. Circadian rhythm of adrenal cortical activity in depression. Arch. Gen. Psychiatry, 1968; 19:672-81.

Gallagher. Adrenocorticol carcinoma in man. The effect of amphenone on individual ketosteroids. J. Clin. Endocrinol., 1958; 18:937-949.

Gower, D.B.; Honour, J.W. Part 1. Steroid catabolism and urinary excretion. Part 2. Biliary excretion and enterohepatic circulation. In: Biochemistry of Steroid Hormones. H.L.J. Makin, ed., Blackwell Scientific Publ.; Oxford, pp. 349-408, 1984.

Jacobsen, M.A.; Fusaro, R.E.; Galmarini, M. et. al. Decreased serum dehydroepiandrosterone is associated with an increased progression of human immunodeficiency virus infection in men with CD-4 cell counts of 200-499. J. Infect. Dis. 1997; 164:864-8.

Jesse, R.L.; Loessner, K.; Eich, D.M. et. al. DHEA inhibits human platelet aggregation in vitro and in vivo. Ann. NY Acad. Sci. 1995; 774:281-90.

Kalimi, M.; Opoku, J.; Lu, R. et. al. Studies on the biochemical action and mechanism of dehydroepiandrosterone. In: The Biologic Role of Dehydroepiandrosterone (DHEA). M. Kalimi, W. Regleson, eds. Walter de Gruyter & Co.:Berlin, pp. 397-404, 1990.

Knudsen, T.T.; Mahesh, V.B. Initiation of precocious sexual maturation in the immature rat treated with dehydroepiandrosterone. Endocrinology 1995; 97:458-68.

Krieger, D.T. Pathophysiology of central nervous system regulation of anterior pituitary function. In: Biology of Brain Dysfunction, Vol. II. Plenum Press:New York, pp. 351-408, 1973.

Lardy, H. Personal communication, 1997.

Lardy, H.; Partridge, B.; Kneer, N. et. al. Ergosteroids: induction of thermogenic enzymes in liver of rats treated with steroids derived from dehydroepiandrosterone. Proc. Nat. Acad. Sci. 1995; 92:6617-6619.

Lieberman, S.; Dorbiner, K.; Hill, B.R.; Fieser, L.F.; Rhoads, C.P. Studies in steroid metabolism. II. Identification and characterization of ketosteroids isolated from urine of healthy and diseased persons. J. Biol. Chem., 1948; 172:263-295.

Lopea, S.A. Lancet 1967; 485-87.

Loria, R.M.; Inge, T.H.; Cook, S.S. et. al. Up-regulation of the immune response and resistance to virus infection with dehydroepiandrosterone (DHEA), In: Hormones, Thermogenesis and Obesity. H. Lardy and F. Stratman, eds. Elsevier: New York, pp. 427-439, 1989.

Loria, R.M.; Inge, T.H.; Cook, S.S. et. al. Protection against acute lethal viral infections with the native steroid dehydroepiandrosterone (DHEA). Jnl. Med. Virol. 1988; 26:301-314.

Marham, P.D.; Salahuddin, S.Z.; Veren, K. et. al. Hydrocortisone and some other hormones enhance the expression of HTLV-111. Int. J. Cancer 1986; 37:67-72.

McLachlin, J.A.; Serkin, C.D. et. al. DHEA modulation of lipopolysaccharide-stimulated monocyte cytotoxicity. J. Immunol. 1996; 157(1):328-35.

McLachlan, J.A.; Serkin, C.D.; Bakouche, O. Dehydroepiandrosterone and androsterone levels in human plasma. Effect of age and sex; day-to-day and diurnal variations. J. Clin. Endrocrinol. Metab. 1957; 17:1051-1062.

Meikle, A.W.; Dorchuk, R.W.; Araneo, B.A. et. al. The presence of a dehydroepiandrosterone-specific receptor binding complex in murine T-cells. J. Steroid Biochem. Molec. Biol. 1992; 42:293-304.

Membreno, L.; Irony, I.; Dere, W. et. al. Andrenocortical function in acquired immunodeficiency syndrome. J. Clin. Endocrinol. Metab. 1987; 65:482-7.

Merril, C.R.; Harrington, M.G.; Sutherland, T. Plasma dehydroepiandrosterone levels in HIV infection [letter]. JAMA 1989; 261:1149.

Merril, C.R. Reduced plasma dehydroepiandrosterone concentrations in HIV infection and Alzheimer's disease. In: The Biologic Role of Dehydroepiandrosterone (DHEA). M. Kalimi, W. Regelson, eds. Walter de Gruyter Co.: Berlin, pp. 101-105, 1990.

Mitchell, L.E.; Sprecher, D.L. et. al. Evidence of an association between DHEAS and nonfatal premature myocardial infarctions in males. Circulation, 1994; 89:91-3.

Morales, A.J.; Nolan, J.J.; Nelson, J.C.; Yen, S.S.C. Effects of replacement dose of dehydroepiandrosterone in men and women of advancing age. J. Clin. Endocrinol. Metab. 1994; 78:1360-67.

Mortola, J.F.; Liu, J.H.; Gillin, J.C. et. al. Pulsatile rhythms of ACTH and cortisol in women with endogenous depression: Evidence for increased ACTH pulse frequency. J. Clin. Endocrinol. Metab. 1987; 65(5):962-8.

Mortola, J.F.; Yen, S.S.C. The effects of oral dehydroepiandrosterone on endocrine-metabolic parameters in postmenopausal women. Jnl. Clin. Endocrinol. and Metab. 1990; 71:696-704.

Mulder, J.W.; Frissen, P.H.J.; Krijnen, P. et. al. DHEA as a predictor for progression to AIDS in asymptomatic HIV-infected men. J. Infect. Dis. 1992; 165:413-18.

Nestler, J.E.; Barlascini, C.O.; Clore, J.N. et. al. Dehydroepiandrosterone reduces serum low density lipoprotein levels and body fat but does not alter insulin sensitivity in normal men. J. Clin. Endocrinol. Metab. 1988; 66:57-61.

Nowata, H.; Tanaka, S.; Takayangi, R. et. al. Aromtase in bone cell: Association with osteoporosis in postmenopausal women. J. Steroid Biochem. Molec. Biol. 1995; 53(1-6):165-74.

Orentreich, N.; Brind, J.L.; Rizer, R.L. et. al. Age changes and sex differences in serum dehydroepiandrosterone sulfate concentrations throughout adulthood. J. Clin. Endocrinol. Metab. 1984; 59:551-555.

Padgett, D.A.; Loria, R.M. In vitro potentiation of lymphocyte activation by dehyrdoepiandrosterone, androstenediol and androstenetriol. Jnl. Immunol. 1994; 153:1544-1552.

Regelson, W.; Kalimi, M.; Loria, R. Dehydroepiandrosterone (DHEA): the precursor steroid. Introductory remarks. In: The Biologic Role of Dehydroepiandrosterone (DHEA). M. Kalimi, W. Regelson, eds. Walter de Gruyter & Co.: Berlin, pp. 1-6, 1990b.

Regelson, W.; Kalimi, M. Dehydroepiandrosterone—the multifunctional steroid. II. Effects on the CNS, cell proliferation, metabolic and vascular, clinical and other effects, Mechanism of Action? Ann. NY Acad. Sci. 1994B; 719:564-75.

Regelson, W.; Loria, R.; Kalimi, M. Hormonal intervention: buffer hormones or state dependency. The role of dehydroepiandrosterone (DHEA): thyroid hormone, estrogens and hypophysectomy in aging. NW Acad. Sci. 1988; 521:260-73.

Riley, V. Psychoneuroendocrine influence on immune competence and neoplasia. Science, 1983; 212:1100-1109.

Roberts, E.; Fitten, L.J. Serum steroid levels in two old men with Alzheimer's disease (AD) before, during and after oral administration of dehydroepiandrosterone (DHEA0. Pregnenolone synthesis may become rate-limiting in aging. In: The Biologic Role of Dehydroepiandrosterone (DHEA). M. Kalimi, W. Regelson, eds. Walter de Gruyter & Co.: Berlin, pp. 43-63, 1990.

Roberts, E.; Fauble, T.J. Oral dehydroepiandrosterone in multiple sclerosis. Results of a phase one, open study. In: The Biologic Role of Dehydroepiandrosterone (DHEA). M. Kalimi, W. Regelson, eds. Walter de Gruyter & Co: Berlin, pp. 81-92, 1990.

Roberts, E.; Fauble, T.J. Oral DHEA in multiple sclerosis. Results of a phase one, open study. In: The Biologic Note of DHEA. Walter de Gruyter & Co., pp. 81-92, 1990.

Rosenfeld, R.S.; Rosenberg, B.J.; Fukushima, D.K. et. al. 24-hour secretory pattern of dehydroisoandrosterone and dehydroisoandrosterone sulfate. J. Clin. Endocrinol. Metab. 1975; 40:850.

Schinazi, R.F.; Eriksson, B.F.H.; Arnold, B. et. al. Effect of dehydroepiandrosterone (DHEA) in lymphocytes and macrophages infected with HIV-1 [abstract MCP 44]. In: Abstracts of the V Intl. Conf. on AIDS, Montreal, 1989.

Schwartz, A.G.; Lewbart, M.L.; Pashko, L.L. Novel dehydroepiandrosterone analogues with enhanced biological activity and reduced side effects in mice and rats. Cancer Res. 1988; 48:4817-22.

Shafogoj, Y.; Opoku, J.; Qureshi, D. et. al. Dehydroepiandrosterone prevents dexamethasone-induced hypertension in rats. Am. J. Physio. 1992; 263:E210-E213.

Sholiton, L.J.; Werk, E.E.; Marnell, R.T. Diurnal variation of adrenocorticol function in non-endocrine disease states. Metabolism 1961; 10:632-46.

Sirianthsinghji, D.J.; Mills, I.H. Concentration patterns of plasma dehydroepiandrosterone, delta-5-androstenediol and their sulphates, testosterone, and cortisol in normal healthy women and in women with anorexia nervosa. Acta. Endocrinol. (Copenhagen) 1985; 108:255-60.

Sonka, J. ACTA Univ. Carol. 1976; 71:146-71.

Svec, F.; Lopez, S.A. Antiglucocorticoid actions of dehydroepiandrosterone and low concentrations in Alzheimer's disease (letter to editor). The Lancet, Dec. 1989; 2:1335-1336.

Tucci, J.R.; Albacet, R.A.; Martin, M.M. Effect of liver disease upon steroid circadian rhythms in man. Gasteroenterol. 1966; 50:637-44.

Van Vollenhoven, R.F.; Engleman, E.G.; McGuire, J.L. An open study of dehydroepiandrosterone in systemic lupus erythematosus. Arthritis and Rheumatism, 1994; 37:1305-10.

Van Vollenhoven, R.F.; Engleman, E.G.; McGuire, J.L. Dehydroepiandrosterone in systemic lupus erythematosus: results of a double-blind, placebo-controlled, randomized clinical trial. Arthritis and Rheumatism, 1995; 38:1826-31.

Vande Wiele, R.L.; Lieberman, S. The metabolism of dehydroisoandrosterone. In: Biological Activities of Steroids in Relation to Cancer. G. Pincus, E.P. Vollmer, eds., Academic Press: New York, pp. 93-110, 1960.

Vande Wiele, R.L.; Macdonald, P.C.; Gurpide, E. et. al. Studies on secretion and interconversation of androgens. Recent Prog. Horm. Res. 1963; 19:275-310.

Villette, J.M.; Bourin, P.; Domel, C. et. al. Circadian variations in plasma levels of hypophyseal, adrenocortical and testicular hormones in men infected with human immunodeficiency virus. Jnl. Clin. Endocrinol. Metab. 1990; 70:572-77.

Villette, J.M.; Bouron, P.; Domel, C. et. al. Circadian variations in plasma levels of hypophyseal, adrenocortical and testicular hormones in women infected with HIV. Jnl. Clin. Endocrinol. Metab. 1990; 70:572-77.

Von Vollenhoven, R.F.; Engelman, E.G.; McGuire, J.L. An open study of DHEA in SLE. Arthritis and Rheum. 1994; 37(9):1305-10.

Welle, S.; Jozefowicz, R.; Statt, M. Failure of dehydroepiandrosterone to influence energy and protein metabolism in humans. Jnl. Clin. Endocrinol. Metab. 1990; 71:1259-64.

Yen, T.T.; Allan, J.A.; Pearson, D.V. et. al. Prevention of obesity in Ayv/a mice by dehydroepiandrosterone. Lipids 1977; 12:409-413.

Yen, S.S.C. The effects of oral DHEA on endocrine metabolic parameters in postmenopausal women. Jnl. Clin. Endocrinol. and Metab. 1990; 71:696-704.

Chapter 4

Faredin, I.; Webb, J.L.; Julesa, M. The in vitro metabolism of dehydroepiandrosterone in human skin. Acta. Medica. Acad., Sci. Hungaricae 1967; 23:169-190.

Gallagher, Adrenocorticol carcinoma in man: the effect of amplerone on individual ketosteroids. J. Clin. Endocrinol. 1958; 18:937-949.

Lardy, H. Personal conversation, 1997.

Marenich, L.P. Testosterone, epitestosterone, androstene-dione and 7-keto- dehydroepiandrostendion excretion in healthy men of different ages. Probl. Endokrinol. (USSR) 1979; 25:28-31.

Parker, L.N. Adrenal Androgens in Clinical Medicine. Academic Press: San Diego, 1989.

Chapter 5

DeLuca, H.F. The Vitamin D Story: a collaborative effort of basic science and clinical medicine. FASEB J. 2:224-236; 1988.

DeLuca, H.F. Remembrance: Discovery of the Vitamin D Endocrine System. Endocrinology, 130:1763, 1992.

DeLuca, H.F. Vitamin D: 1993, Nutrition Today, 28:#6, 1993.

Acknowledgements

It is amazing to me how much help I needed to make this book possible. I am truly grateful to everyone who supported this manuscript through its formative stages.

A special thanks to Lois Olson whose extraordinary technical skills made this manuscript come alive on paper, and to Donna Good whose expertise in editing and organization made the book presentable.

I am indebted to Dr. Henry Lardy and Dr. Hector DeLuca for granting me interviews and tolerating my many questions. I also thank them for their vision, particularly Dr. Lardy, for without his enthusiasm for DHEA derivatives and their potential, portions of this book would not have evolved.

Thanks also to Linda Ahrndt, my nurse of many years, who has been a trusted friend to me and my patients. She shares my passion for treating the physical and emotional needs of patients and understands often better than I, the holistic needs of sick people. Together we have embraced the principles of an integrated health model as we watched our patients improve with both allopathic and complementary medical treatments.

My very special gratitude though goes to my wife Connie, who has never stopped believing in my aspirations. Her support during the creation of this manuscript was invaluable to me and certainly made the process of writing my first book more enjoyable for both of us.

Lastly and most importantly, I am truly humbled and

forever grateful to all my patients who have placed their trust in my skills and judgement. I am honored to have had the chance to be their physician. The very concept for this book would not have occurred without my patients first introducing me to the benefits of complementary medicine. I am forever indebted to their insight and passion for a healthy and vital lifestyle.

Other publications of **Advanced Research Press, Inc.**
150 Motor Pkwy., Suite 210, Hauppauge, NY 11788

All Natural **MUSCULAR DEVELOPMENT** magazine brings its
readers the very best and latest scientific information on strength
training, physique development, nutrition, health and fitness in an
entertaining and contemporary format: 12 issues – $29.88
(50% off cover price)
To order call: 1-888-841-8007

*OPTIMUM SPORTS NUTRITION, **Your Competitive Edge**,* by Dr.
Michael Colgan – a complete guide to the nutritional requirements
of athletes. 562 pages – soft cover $24.95.
To order call: 1-888-841-8007

*PERIODIZATION BREAKTHROUGH! **The Ultimate Training
System*** by Drs. Fleck and Kraemer. A straight forward explanation
of periodized training. An essential system for successful strength
training. 182 pages – hardcover $19.95
To order call: 1-888-841-7996

MUSCLE MEALS By John Romano. A cookbook for bodybuilders
and all athletes featuring a delicious array of easy-to-prepare
energy-packed low-fat meals. Written by culinary expert, TV chef
on ESPN's American Muscle Meals. 24 pages – hardcover $19.95
To order call: 1-888-841-7996

MIKE MENTZER (new advanced)
HIGH INTENSITY TRAINING PROGRAM. A series of 4 audio-
taped lectures, each approximately 50 minutes, by Mike Mentzer,
Mr. Universe Champion, student and master of the art of
bodybuilding covering these topics:

        Tape 1   The Logical Path to Successful Bodybuilding
        Tape 2   Fundamentals of Muscular Development
        Tape 3   Bodybuilding Nutrition De-mystified
        Tape 4   The Man and the Controversy

Included with these tapes is a 40 page High Intensity Training
Program Guide. $39.95.
To order call: 1-888-841-7996